M000287496

A THERAPIST'S GARDEN
Using Plants to Revitalize Your Spirit

Erik Keller

Cover and plate illustrations by Rosana Chinchilla
Spot illustrations by Juana Chinchilla Keller

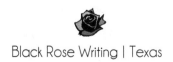

Black Rose Writing | Texas

©2022 by Wapiti LLC
All rights reserved. No part of this book may be reproduced, stored in a retrieval system or transmitted in any form or by any means without the prior written permission of the publishers, except by a reviewer who may quote brief passages in a review to be printed in a newspaper, magazine or journal.

The author grants the final approval for this literary material.

First printing

Some names and identifying details have been changed to protect the privacy of individuals.

ISBN: 978-1-68433-914-3
PUBLISHED BY BLACK ROSE WRITING
www.blackrosewriting.com

Printed in the United States of America
Suggested Retail Price (SRP) $19.95

A Therapist's Garden is printed in Georgia

*As a planet-friendly publisher, Black Rose Writing does its best to eliminate unnecessary waste to reduce paper usage and energy costs, while never compromising the reading experience. As a result, the final word count vs. page count may not meet common expectations.

Further praise for
A Therapist's Garden

A Therapist's Garden eloquently demonstrates that nurturing plant life and immersing oneself in the seasonal cycles of nature is often the best prescription for health and well being.

—Matt Mattus, author of *Mastering the Art of Flower Gardening* and the award-winning gardening blog *Growing with Plants*

A wonder-filled book of the hidden miracles of therapeutic gardening. *A Therapist's Garden* captures Erik Keller's many years of experience with inspiring tales of success with special-needs children and plants. A joy to read!

—Sal Gilbertie, author and owner Gilbertie's Herb Gardens, one of the largest organic herb growers in the United States

This engaging book is filled with month-by-month chapters of delightful stories from Erik's many years of teaching horticultural therapy. *A Therapist's Garden* has many useful gardening tips and projects bringing the therapeutic benefits of plants into clients' lives.

—Marc Thoma, author of Urban Gardening for Beginners and Herb Gardening for Beginners, tranquilurbanhomestead.com

A Therapist's Garden is a timeless yet timely account of how plants and gardening have the power to influence, heal and possibly transform lives. Over years and seasons, Erik Keller weaves together deeply personal stories and practical information for all who are interested in learning how horticulture is an unparalleled therapeutic medium.

—Phyllis D'Amico, HTM, Program Coordinator, Horticultural Therapy, The New York Botanical Garden

I dedicate this book to my daughters, Kathryn and Sarah, who made me young at heart, and to my grandchildren, Charlotte, Charlie, and Olivia who are keeping me that way.

CONTENTS

ACKNOWLEDGMENTS

A book like this has many participants to whom I am grateful. First and foremost are the clients, friends, and family who have given me the privilege to help them and become a healing presence in their lives. Much of this is via the organizations that have allowed me the opportunity to work with their clients. They include Ann's Place (Danbury, Connecticut), Meadow Ridge (Redding, Connecticut), and Green Chimneys (Brewster, New York). I would also like to thank Reagan Rothe of Black Rose Writing for giving me the opportunity to publish my story.

Any book requires guidance from a trusted group of readers. In my case they include Susan Baker, Phyllis D'Amico, Wilda Hayes, and John Reiner. A special callout goes to one of my early mentors, Tracy Chamberlin, who came up with the title, *A Therapist's Garden*. Extra thanks goes to Theodore Sklar whose relentless and careful editing and suggestions early on ultimately made the book much more focused and readable. And finally, Ellen Lewis is a remarkable editor who took my final draft and with deft knowledge and a delicate touch polished it to a fine finish.

The cover and much of the artwork inside is a labor of love by illustrator Rosana Chinchilla. She has captured the essence of not only the seasonal change in the gardens I inhabit but the joy of those who share them with me.

And my wife, Juana, has been instrumental in getting this book published. She was my first and most encouraging reader, and she has taken this project to heart as her own, also creating a portion of the art for the pages. This book would be much the worse without her gentle and loving counsel, encouragement, and keen memory. I am forever grateful for her assistance.

A THERAPIST'S GARDEN

PREFACE

At the entrance of a drab, red-bricked building hidden in the woods, I push the buzzer on the intercom, identifying myself and the person I am there to see. A crackly, static-laden voice acknowledges my request, and after a minute the large, gray steel entry door swings open toward me. I am led down a concrete stairwell with beige block walls and through another locked steel door. I then walk along a stark hallway lined with gray doors, each having a tiny glass window at eye level. Turning left, I exit via a windowless metal door into a small yard surrounded by a galvanized chain-link fence topped with barbed wire. In the middle of an untended mat of weeds and grass sits an empty but magnificent greenhouse.

"Do you think you can help us use it to grow plants?" asks one pony-tailed girl standing within a group.

Dressed in white sweatshirts, black sweatpants, and cheap white sneakers, the girls appear sad, hurt, embarrassed, and scared that they are trapped in a juvenile detention center. They are just children. But after a few weeks, these morose detainees are transformed into happy teens after we clean up the greenhouse and start to build a garden that they will care for and own.

Over two decades ago, that was my introduction to the healing power and potential for joy that horticultural therapy can deliver to people. I continue to see it daily.

In many ways, we are all horticultural therapists whenever we bring a bundle of freshly cut flowers to a loved one in the hospital or a fresh rosemary plant to a chef who needs this aromatic herb for a favorite poultry dish. The patient trapped in a hospital bed, even if unable to speak, lights up at the sight of roses, daisies, or chrysanthemums being placed on a nearby table. The chef breathes in the fresh fragrance of rosemary while tenderly selecting the branches for a recipe, releasing the essential oils from the soft needles. There is happiness and peace in these simple acts.

Before I retired from working in the corporate world, I often took solace in my garden after a stressful workday. When my mother was dealing with my father's treatment for lung cancer, it was side trips to nurseries that gave her momentary respite and calm as she smelled the flowers at hand and thought back to her mother's garden in Donora, Pennsylvania. These simple therapies are incredibly effective.

I started my training in horticultural therapy by joining the Master Gardener program at the University of Connecticut (UCONN). Every state in the U.S. and eight Canadian provinces sponsor similar programs. In the U.S. they do so through land-grant universities and Cooperative Extension Services, where non-professionals have the opportunity to obtain a wide swath of experience and lessons from university instructors and professors on gardening and horticulture. In the UCONN program that I joined, my classmates and I took seven-hour courses once a week for four months, took tests, volunteered on a gardening hotline answering questions concerning plants, volunteered for a community project, and then took a comprehensive final exam at the end of the year of study.

Master Gardener classes are split into many different areas: trees, shrubs, flowers, soil, propagation, disease, insects, and more. Students attending these programs possess varying skills, though most have spent many a year on their knees weeding gardens and tending plants. A few are landscape professionals who seek the certification as a feather in their well-worn and soiled baseball caps. While taking classes, we were instructed on the basics of botany and gardening, which helped me discover how much I still needed to learn, such as how beneficial it can be to know the Latin names for plants. For the plants that play a part in this book, I have used common names but also have supplied the Latin at first mention in each chapter. An index of plant names is included as well.

A few years later as I pondered retirement, I leafed through a course catalog from the New York Botanical Garden (NYBG). My wife had been taking courses in botanical illustration; in the back of the catalog was a section on horticultural therapy. I thought back to my experiences working in the detention center and comforting my mother as cancer was taking my father away from her. Something clicked—this course was what I needed for the next phase of my life.

Immediately, I started to take classes for my certification in horticultural therapy, learning how to use gardening to help clients overcome cognitive, emotional, social, and physical challenges. I learned how to design therapeutic gardens. I was taught how to create plant-centric activities using all of the five senses. And just as important, I discovered how to create programs with a small budget, as horticultural therapy is often underfunded.

Obtaining a certification in horticultural therapy forced me to stretch my skills and emotions. Being a good therapist is not about growing the best-looking plant, it is about using plants and Nature to help a client better cope with trying issues. The most useful aspect about the NYBG program was an internship of one hundred hours working side-by-side with experienced horticultural therapists and their clients. Understanding the difference between the pistil and stamen of a flower is important but pales in comparison to connecting with a client and evoking a smile.

For over twenty years, I have had the privilege to help people of all ages in a variety of facilities in the New York metropolitan area. My clients have included special-needs children, incarcerated youths, family members, seniors with physical and cognitive challenges, and cancer patients and survivors. Working with them, I have seen how horticultural therapy can change people's lives in a positive fashion. I have fictionalized the names of clients in the following pages to preserve their confidentiality, but most of the facilities where I have practiced are identified by name.

The organization of this book follows that of the calendar, January to December. It also takes place in New England, thus readers who live in other areas may not recognize the timing of seasonal change as it is written. Its stories cover two decades of time, from the past to the present and back. This is most obvious in the sections including my granddaughter, Charlotte, who jumps from an infant to a young child to a toddler. In addition, in each month I offer a horticultural therapy craft as well as an outing for readers to consider. Each story attempts to show different approaches and tools and how they address the varying needs of my clients. I would like to share some of their stories, as well as mine, with you.

Erik Keller
Ridgefield, CT
February 2022

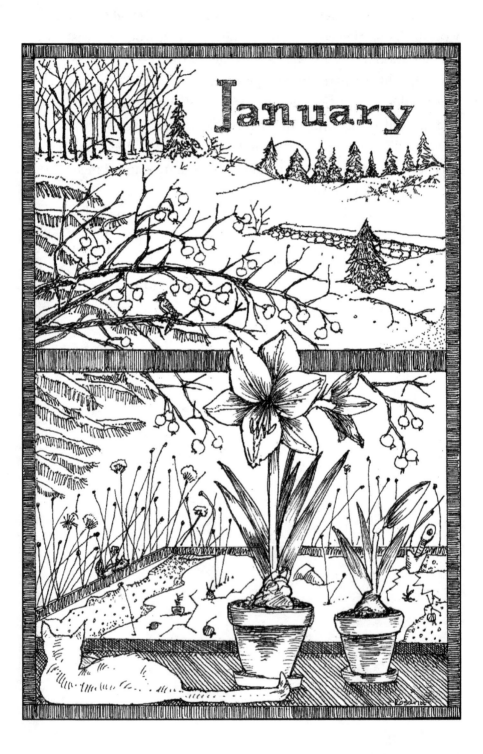

JANUARY: A COLD BEGINNING

The start of the year, January, has much to do with entrances. In Latin, January is Ianuarius; ianua is Latin for door. The mythical Roman god Janus is the god of beginnings and transitions. And it is a transition for those of us living in the North. With the seasonal holidays behind us, the warmth and greening of Spring is months away. But there are bright spots and opportunities to enjoy the otherwise cold weather, as well as the garden.

LET'S KILL THE RAT!

We are still harvesting lettuce greens (*Lactuca sativa*) in the Children's Garden even though the hoop houses—temporary structures that have been sheltering our garden rows since early Fall—are blanketed in snow. The Children's Garden is part of Green Chimneys, a therapeutic school and treatment center for children with special needs in Brewster, New York. With the prospect of a warming weekend, we decide to remove the snow from the hoops to see if our luck continues to hold.

My first charge, David, will help me in this task. He is looking forward to going outside, as it is an ideal day for early January, sunny and windless with a temperature a little under forty degrees. Later in the day, even in this chill, it should be warm enough to pick greens. Reaching the garden entrance, we attempt to open the padlock on the garden gate, but it is frozen and we must try to enter via a side gate that doesn't have a lock. We get in easily.

The garden appears quiet and lifeless. Everything is coated with a layer of smooth, white snow, marred only by the few animals that have scurried around the landscape leaving indistinguishable footprints. Dried heads of dill *(Anethum graveolens)* as well as those of a few sunflowers *(Helianthus annuus)* poking their heads high are the only visual signs of past crops. The hoop houses appear as a series of undulating, bright white speed bumps in the distance.

The sound of crunching snow follows us as we create imperfections, paths on our way toward the shed to retrieve shovels. David strains a bit at the cold and the strength required to swing open the shed door, which is blocked by drifts of snow. The door gives way eventually and a white moth flutters out, not realizing that its prior home is a much better place to stay. Grabbing a set of shovels, we start to clear the snow off the hoops, which are covered with Agribon, a white protective outdoor fabric. The snow is starting to melt from the sun and slides off in icy clumps when coaxed. We are careful in removing the cloth's frozen covering so as not to rip it.

Soon the snow is off and we remove the Agribon to see how well the corn salad *(Valerianella locusta)* and mustard greens (*Brassica juncea*) are doing. Suddenly something scampers, going into hiding. It is a rat and is as surprised as we are. The hoop house is not a bad place to be in Winter if you are a rat. It contains leftover greens, drops of water from the melting snow, and a warmer nest than a rat would have under or in a log. It reminds me of the rat Templeton in E. B. White's delightful children's story *Charlotte's Web*, but in this case, the creature is scared, now running around looking for a new place to hide, finding only hard ground or soft snow to tunnel through.

"Let's kill it!" yells David, excited by this discovery.

"With what?" I say, remembering a past episode at my house. My wife had said that if I had owned a gun, I would have been able to shoot the rat that had taken up residence under our bed while we were on vacation. "We have shovels," replies David.

"Let's just leave it alone, because we could hurt it rather than kill it, which would be heartless," I reply. I have never been a hunter of animals, and the idea of flailing around in the snow with a shovel and a rat has all the makings of a cruel disaster. We leave the rat and greens in their places, put back the Agribon fabric, and start to clean off other hoops for the rest of our time together.

My next student, Charles, is interested to see if the carrots (*Daucus carota* subsp. *sativus)* are still growing. The sun is higher in the sky and some of the greens that were uncovered earlier have rehydrated. They can be picked now, though the ground is rock hard. Pulling off the Agribon draped over the hoops, I notice a brown spider that is clinging to the underside of the cloth.

I think it is dead, but after a few minutes it starts to twitch and move around. I feel bad that I disturbed it, as it will need to find another place to settle in for Winter. Even during this unforgiving time of year, there is life all around us to appreciate.

While I ponder the spider's ultimate fate, Charles is trying to dig out a carrot in an adjacent raised bed. The ground is still very frozen, even though the carrot tops are green and appear fresh. They are tempting—the frozen soil causes the starch in carrots to be converted to sugar, thus making them increasingly sweet as Winter stretches on.

Charles, however, is now very frustrated at his inability to harvest a carrot. I tell him to keep trying and be patient, but in less than a minute he is on the verge of tears because of his perceived failure.

"Charles, let's look for a carrot at the edge of the garden beds. If it's close enough to the boards, perhaps the sun has thawed some of the soil that's holding it in place," I suggest. Charles wipes his eyes and nose with his glove and stops sniffling, nodding his head in agreement.

After hunting around a bit, we find such a carrot and I am able to insert a trowel between it and the boards of the raised bed. I wiggle the trowel and then give the carrot a tug. No good. I then push the trowel through the soil on the other side of the carrot. More wiggling and the soil starts to move. Charles grabs it. He pulls. It comes out of the soil intact.

"I got a carrot!" Charles yells as his emotions flip from despair to delight. While he is tempted, he doesn't eat it immediately. "I'm going to bring the carrot home so my mom can make a healthy soup with it for my family," he says. "I'll tell her that I picked it from the garden today. She'll never believe me." We put away our tools and lock up the shed. Walking back to his classroom, Charles smiles and protects his carrot, brushing bits of ice and soil off its surface before putting it into his pocket.

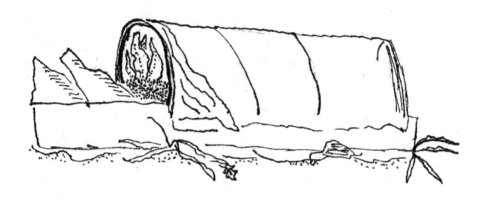

SEEDING DESIRE

January is a month where days can be brightened by unexpected discoveries. At this time of year, I am quick to collect the daily mail to devour the seed and plant catalogs that arrive. They all bring a smile to my face as I sit in front of the wood stove with a cup of coffee or tea, looking out upon the snow and the birds feasting on sunflower seeds and suet.

For my clients at Ann's Place, a cancer support facility in Danbury, Connecticut, these mailings open a planning window that portends warm breezes and fragrant scents. As clients wait for class to start, still shivering from being outside, I walk around them giving each a seed or plant catalog.

"While you all may think that Spring is very far away, it's actually a good time to think about what you want to put in your garden later this year," I start. "Think about it. Your space is now devoid of weeds and deciduous leaves. You have a clean pallet. Think about what you would like to see. Look in the catalogs for some of your favorite plants and the possibilities that a warmer season will afford you."

I share with the class a wide selection of catalogs, including Johnny's Select Seeds, Territorial, Burpee, Bluestone Perennials, John Scheepers, Fedco, Norse, Park Seed, Seed Savers Exchange, and

Baker's Creek. I let my clients sit and absorb their contents. Questions crop up quickly.

"Where do you order your seeds?"

"How early should we start flowers from seed?"

"Could I start a microgreen garden now?"

"How big are the bushes they send you and will the deer eat them?"

Everyone starts looking over each other's shoulders at alternative catalogs, sharing pages and favorites. Smartphones come out and pictures are snapped. A few ask if they can start tomatoes (*Solanum lycopersicum*) soon, but I tell them no, they need to wait for warmer weather and longer days. They don't seem to mind, and I smile to myself that for at least this moment in their day my clients are sitting in a brighter and warmer place.

JANUARY CRAFT: GROW SOME SPROUTS

*While few may think of January as a time to sow a garden, there are many things that can be planted indoors, even in the confines of a small apartment. When my wife and I were newlyweds, our love of stir-fry made us farmers of a continuous supply of mung bean (*Vigna radiata*) sprouts.*

Growing new plants in the dead of Winter is one of the best ways to shake off the chill of the season; a handful of mung beans is a simple beginning. There are many ways to plant them, but my wife, Juana, and I soaked the beans overnight, drained them, and put them in a mason jar, leaving them uncovered. We placed the jar under a bookshelf, and every day we rinsed the beans with water, leaving them wet. Within a couple of days, we were ready to harvest sprouts for our mostly vegetarian meals.

POTTING UP

Amaryllises *(Hippeastrum)* are sold and marketed in stores as Christmas bulbs, but they are one of the plants that sustains me beyond that holiday. Though I buy new bulbs every few years, most of my blooms are from ones I have kept for a long time. Many people do not realize that these tropical bulbs will reflower year after year. My challenge has always been to get prior years' plants to bloom at Christmas; there never seems to be enough of a cooling period for them after Summer. After a while I stopped trying and decided that I will just pot up a few bulbs every other week in the New Year so that I have big blossoms for the entire Winter.

Bringing a few pots up from the basement, I notice that their soils, along with those of my Christmas cacti *(Schlumbergera bridgesii)*, are hard with whitish minerals. They need larger pots and new soil. With a big potting job in front of me, the best helper I can get to mix the soil is my granddaughter, Charlotte.

Charlotte has been helping me with tactile chores ever since she was five months old. When I make bread she loves to stick her hands into the dough, mixing it as best she can. Charlotte's bread kneading skills will come in handy while I hydrate the soil.

I have learned the hard way to always wet your soil first before potting up, so that your carefully placed seeds and plants stay where you put them rather than float up or tilt badly; it also tamps down dust, preventing inhalation. For Charlotte, mixing soil and water lets her get her hands good and muddy.

An earthy smell of life emerges as I pour the soil into a small mixing tub. Scents of pine and composted cow manure fill the kitchen as we knead the mixture and start to add water.

Charlotte quickly jettisons a small spoon I give her (like many of the children I have worked with over the years) preferring to use both her hands to squeeze and squish the soil. Her hands disappear beneath chunks of soil, leaving a soft, uniform loam that coats her forearms and T-shirt. When we add more water she grabs the remaining chunks, breaks them up, and creates muddy balls that she smiles and giggles about.

The correct consistency of a wet soil mix is one where you can create and squeeze a firm ball without water dripping from it. We are close to the ideal proportions, though Charlotte wants to add a lot more water. I am able to stop her from doing that by telling her to keep swirling her hands in the tub so we can make mud pies later. She agrees.

After we obtain the right soil consistency, I try to get Charlotte to help me put soil in the pots, but she is too interested in enveloping her arms in the mixture. Soon she is covered hand to armpit in a patina of white perlite, slivers of compost, and chunks of peat moss. She dunks her arms in the watering can to clean them but then immediately reintroduces soil tattoos to her arms by rolling them in the mixing tub.

We first remove the Christmas cacti from their pots and strip them of their soil leaving bare roots. Charlotte then takes handfuls of small pebbles and places them in the bottom of the pots so there will be lots of drainage. We take sand from a separate container and combine it with the hydrated soil to make a lighter cactus mix. She giggles again as the rocks and sand sometimes stick to her hands and she needs to brush them off. We then place the roots on top of the pebbles and the soil around the sides of each cactus.

We soon have a group of new pots ready to be placed by the window. The amaryllises are next, but Charlotte is hungry and demands a treat before we continue—hot chocolate and cookies. It seems fair payment.

FRESH SMELLS, COLD TEMPERATURES

Going green is challenging now in New England as there is a dearth of fresh local material. But a little advance planning goes a long way toward making you believe that the bees are buzzing nearby and gnats are biting your arms.

Over a dozen clients fill the art room of clients at Ann's Place to create fragrant sachets. To get us in the right frame of mind for the class, I pass around lemon geranium (*Pelargonium crispum*) and rosemary *(Salvia rosmarinus)* plants that I had brought inside last Fall for this class. We start to talk about smells and which scents are favorites as the plants are passed around. Lavender *(Lavandula angustifolia)* and rose (*Rosa*) rise to the top of the list.

"By rubbing the leaves, you transfer the oils of the plants onto your fingers, and your fingers retain the smells that the oils express," I say. "Use your right hand for one plant and your left for the other so you don't mix the oils and confuse the associated smells." As the plants move between clients so do their expressions—delight, confusion, peaceful remembrance. The fresh scents energize my clients in unexpected, positive ways. But not always.

Last year, an elderly man wearing a tattered sports jacket attended a sachet class. Bill had just lost his wife to cancer and was looking for solace and comfort. His face was drawn and he looked down toward his hands resting on the table, saying little as the group gathered. Bill wanted to make a sachet in remembrance of his loved one. As he sampled the different oils, tears came to his eyes suddenly as he placed down one of the vials. "My wife loved lavender and this smells just like the flowers she used to pick and put in a vase in the hallway," Bill said. "I'm sorry." He got up and left. Bill never attended any of my classes again. I was hoping that this class would not elicit a similar response from any of my clients.

"There are two types of oils, essential and fragrant," I explain, starting the class. "Essential oils are the actual oils collected from plants. Fragrant oils are their chemically produced equivalents. In aromatherapy, you always use essential oils as they are natural. Most of the oils we're using are essential oils."

I point out the few fragrant oils in my collection and pick up the vial holding rose oil. "Now the reason why we're using a fragrant oil for rose is that its essential counterpart is very expensive. Most fragrant rose oils are around five to seven dollars for a one-ounce vial like this one. Guess how much that would cost if it were essential?"

The highest anyone guesses is seventy-five dollars. The reality is closer to three hundred.

"We don't have that kind of budget here," I say. Everyone laughs.

With that, my clients start their mixing of spices, herbs, and oils to create a fragrant filling for a sachet. I remind them to be cautious and use only one or two drops of each oil at a time so they may sense the nuances of their concoctions.

As fragrant and essential oil vials pass between clients, Nancy becomes attached to the one holding the French vanilla oil. "This is wonderful," she says as she inhales again and again and again. "I really like this." She is reluctant to share it with anyone else. Some have a difficult time choosing between all the oils and herbs. Others make a bee line to a perceived favorite. A few go overboard with a particular scent.

"This just smells of lemon. Everything else is masked," I tell one client upon smelling her mixture.

"But that is exactly what I want," Katlin replies.

"Can I do anything with this to cut back the smell?" asks April about a sachet that overwhelms with the scent of rosemary. Its aroma can be perceived five feet away.

"I think you went a bit overboard. There isn't much you can do."

Weeks later April returns to class saying how happy she is with her rosemary sachet as it remains in her car and its scent is intact. "Every time I enter the car, it smells so fresh. I love it."

JANUARY OUTING:
SEARCH FOR CREATURES GREAT AND SMALL

Though a thick coating of snow and ice seems intimidating, active life abounds in the outdoors. Many birds do not migrate, and the colorful blue jay is easily identifiable perched on a leafless tree. Bluebirds and cardinals also go about challenging the jay as the most colorful during this gray time of year as they hide in the branches of a nearby evergreen tree.

On warmer days, squirrels scamper up and down trees looking for food, or perhaps are afflicted with a rodent's version of insomnia. Footprints of other *creatures are spotted through the fresh snow. Mouse pathways and tunnels swirl over a space in seemingly mad circles. Occasional rabbit tracks make their way across the ground, and larger imprints of deer hoofs make a line from one safe spot to another. A few birds rest firm on a crabapple (*Malus*) tree then fly over to the winterberry (*Ilex* verticillata*) to sample their shriveled fruits. While most vegetation is dormant, more animals than we think are not.*

COLORS OF SPRING

I try to lighten the mood of clients at Ann's Place by focusing on bright colors and living plants. A class on pressed-flower arrangements meets at least half of that aim, removing my clients from a snow-covered landscape by transporting them into a colorful oasis of garden blooms. To start, I show them samples that Juana has made in postcard-sized picture frames. One is a simple collection of violet and yellow violas (*Viola tricolor*) that overlap each other. The vibrancy of the colors surprises them.

"These are a couple of years old," I start. "You may be surprised to see how long they can keep their colors." My clients are excited to get started.

Online sellers have a wide array of pressed and colored flowers that can be acquired easily. So like a black-jack dealer in Vegas, I deal out cellophane-wrapped sheets of dried and flattened daisies (*Bellis perennis*), baby's breath (*Gypsophila paniculata*), ferns (*Tracheophyta*), chrysanthemums (*Chrysanthemum*), violets (*Viola sororia*), and many other flowers. Every color, size, and texture are offered: blue, yellow, red, green, purple, white, fuzzy, smooth, tiny, large. I may have overwhelmed my clients.

"Where did you get these?"

"Pass me the violets, please."

"Do you have roses?"

Everyone looks to grab samples. I need to slow things down.

"You can buy dried flowers like this, but the good news is that in a few months we can all start saving flowers and drying them ourselves," I say. And with that I show everyone my flower press with samples taken last Summer. A flower press can be as simple as a large book, or it can be a slightly more complex device. Mine is a series of paper and cardboard sheets held together with wooden covers and thumbscrews. I had gathered Queen-Anne's lace (*Daucus carota*), ferns, violas, roses, herbs, and many other flowers from my garden. The shapes and the delicate nature of my pressed posies intrigue all.

"How did you do that? Are we going to build a flower press?" asks Mary. "Yes, but we'll wait until Summer so we can press flowers from our garden here," I reply.

"Why did some of your flowers lose their color?" asks Susan. "Some flowers keep their colors better than others," I explain. "And some people use more complex techniques than I attempt to help make a difference." Few now notice the blowing wind and cold outside. They have entered their own virtual flower gardens.

To get clients started, I suggest that everyone should first decide the colors of the background paper and picture frame they want to use. For instance, to show off a white daisy, a light blue paper could be best, but that color needs to be selected in conjunction with the tone of the picture frame. Next, designs need to be organized and laid out. This way substitutions and changes can be made easily before committing to a final design.

"Everyone should have a set of tweezers to help pick up and arrange the flowers, otherwise you can easily tear them," I say. "After you finish arranging, I'll explain the next steps."

My clients start to organize their flowers. While there is a bit of cross talk, everyone is absorbed in the design and selection of paper, frame, and flowers. Their gazes vacillate between the packets of flowers and their emerging creations. The room remains uncharacteristically silent while they concentrate as would a precision craftsman working on a delicate creation. Italian composer Antonio Vivaldi's classic violin concerto *The Four Seasons* plays in the background.

"Now that you have designed your picture, get a glue stick and apply glue to your paper where you want a flower to remain. Place the flower down with your tweezers and then tap the flower with the other end of the tweezers. This way you don't get excess glue on your fingers or the plant," I say. "And when you finish, let me know and I'll put them in the frames for you."

They glue their creations together carefully. Some use more glue than needed and are forced to redo their designs, but most approach the task with the same concentration as before. Once a design is complete, I frame it deftly. When the last frame is placed on the last picture, I line up all the designs next to each other for a picture. Everyone expresses amazement at how pretty the arrangements turned out. With that they collect their creations and coats and depart to drive home in the snow.

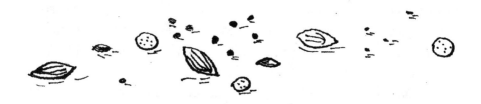

WHITTLING TRUST

Though the snow is not even close to melting and the wood stove in my house has been blasting continuously, we have started seeding early Spring plants in the greenhouse near the Children's Garden. The temperature has not gone north of twenty degrees for over a week, so going outside with children is not possible. The greenhouse, however, is a fine place to be on a sunny day in Winter as it is deliciously toasty and humid. The musty smell of plants is a welcome contrast to the dry, cold air outside or that of a heated, barren classroom.

The job for today is to plant at least two trays each of coleus (*Plectranthus scutellarioides*), pansies (*Viola tricolor* var. *hortensis*), dusty miller (*Jacobaea maritima*), and geraniums (*Pelargonium*). As my first student Maria mixes the appropriate soil and places it into the seedling trays, I think our goal will be relatively simple. Wrong! I open the packet of coleus seeds and suddenly see and remember how tiny they are. I attempt to pick one up, but my stubby digits make it impossible for me. Even Maria, who has the long, delicate fingers of a piano player, is not successful.

I should have considered this aspect of the job before we started and retrieved the hand seeder from the shed to help us with this tedious chore. But I didn't, so I need to come up with an alternative approach as Maria is becoming increasingly frustrated. I then remember my Swiss Army knife. Rarely a day goes by without a use for this essential tool, but I only notice how much I need it when I forget to place it in my pants pocket. Fortunately, it is there when I reach for it.

I need to be extra careful with it when working with the children. The main blade on the knife is very thin and sharp. It has a small groove where you place your fingernail to pull it out from the body of the knife. This groove, in fact, is an ideal size to hold a tiny seed.

"Okay, Maria, this is what we are going to do. Use this Popsicle stick to move a seed over to the blade and place it in the groove. Then move the knife slowly over to the tray and place the seed into the soil."

Maria was indifferent initially to the planting of seeds, but when she sees that she will be able to wield my knife, she becomes very attentive. I show her how to hold the knife, reminding her to never place her fingers next to the blade. For the next forty-five minutes, we work together planting coleus seeds, Maria wielding the knife and me the Popsicle stick. We are not very productive but we work well together. Maria is typically an impatient child, but letting her use my knife motivates her to focus on this task much longer than she would have otherwise.

My next student, Tony, is a different matter. Tony has a difficult time controlling himself and sitting still. Exiting the school, Tony is his typical jittery self. I'm not sure if I should let him use my knife. Maria finished planting the coleus seeds and now the geraniums need to be planted. These seeds are a little larger than the coleus seeds, and Tony has small enough fingers to grab them. I tell him to pick up the seeds and plant them carefully while I use my knife to plant seeds. That way we can work together.

Tony eyes my knife and asks, "Do you know how to whittle?"

"Sure I do. I learned how when I was around your age." Tony is quiet for a bit and then says that he does not know how to whittle. "Would you teach me?" he asks sheepishly.

I am worried about this as Tony's personality can swing without warning. Trusting him with a knife is probably a bad idea. But he is insistent and earnest in his desire to use my knife, so I construct a test.

"Tony, if you can seed these three rows carefully and precisely, I'll show you how to whittle." I think if he can control his motions well enough to accomplish this task, he can whittle safely while closely supervised. Tony agrees.

He then displays a behavior I have never seen from him before. He quickly albeit carefully seeds three rows of geraniums. Typically it would have taken him the entire session to do this task; with the potential reward of whittling lessons, it takes but a few minutes.

I get a Popsicle stick and illustrate to him how to whittle wood and the importance of the angle between the wood and the blade of the knife. "The key to whittling, Tony, is to control the angle of the blade, which affects how deeply it cuts into the wood. But you also need to be careful with the blade and keep your fingers away from it. You are always pushing the blade away from your hand." Tony nods as I show him how to use the knife with a few simple strokes.

I close the blade and give Tony the knife; he holds it awkwardly. I then sit behind him in another chair. I reach around, cradling his hands within mine, and open the knife so together we can shave off a few slivers of wood. Tony is happy and excited at what he is able to do with this new tool. We practice a few more times together and then I let Tony go on his own, but I stay behind him, watchful in case anything unsafe happens. Like all beginners, he has a hard time regulating the depth of the cut and the angle of the blade. He soon turns the stick into slivers.

"Can we make something?" Tony asks. I nod yes and draw the outline of a canoe on another Popsicle stick. He needs to carve out the center of the stick to create his watercraft. He likes the idea of whittling a canoe and starts to work, with me supervising from behind.

He lets his hands slip uncomfortably close to the blade, which causes me to pull them back before his first stroke. "Tony, you need to keep your hands behind the blade. If you don't, I must take the knife away." Tony agrees and starts carving slowly. Correcting him in the past has often brought a retort, but now he takes my advice. He quietly and carefully works on his canoe with slow and deliberate strokes. When finished, his boat looks more like a speedboat than a canoe, but it doesn't matter. He is pleased with it.

We spend the rest of our time together seeding rows of geraniums. Tony finishes the entire tray quickly and without incident. As I walk him to lunch, his face is framed with a big grin and he can't wait to show off his speedboat to his classmates and teacher. I took a chance letting Tony use my knife, but I thought it was worth the risk given how closely I was supervising him and his positive response. It permanently changed our working relationship for the better.

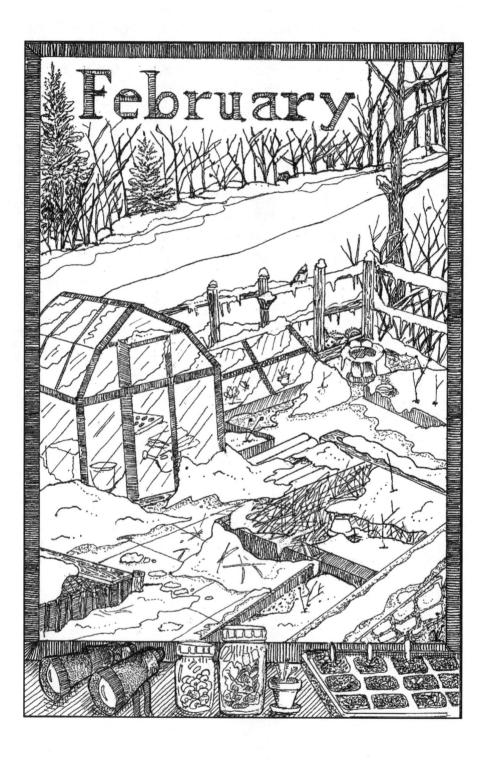

FEBRUARY: COPING WITH CABIN FEVER

The full moon that rises in February is called either the Snow Moon or the Hunger Moon. The moniker Snow Moon seems obvious to most people though the alternate Hunger Moon may not. Centuries ago, if crops were poor in Fall, or the harvest not protected from vermin in Winter, people could run out of sustenance in February, when nourishment to gather is sparse. This is still true, unfortunately, in many parts of the Northern Hemisphere at this time of year.

Many of us don't face that hardship as we can enjoy blueberries this month from South America. Our bigger potential issue is boredom, as the unfulfilled desire to get out of the house and enjoy the outside builds through Winter. Relief often comes when an episodic, fleeting warm spell hits New England and temperatures soar. People dust off shorts and sneakers to take advantage of the respite, before Winter winds and freezing precipitation return for weeks to come.

YOU ARE COLD AND HEARTLESS

"Be mindful of how you organize a flower bouquet," I counsel a group of clients. "You might not realize what you're saying. For instance, a bouquet of hydrangeas (*Hydrangea*) tells someone that they are cold and heartless. Almond (*Prunus dulcis*) blossoms convey stupidity, and a Lenten rose (*Helleborus orientalis*) implies scandal." My clients are shocked.

"On the other hand a red rose (*Rosa*) is passionate love, ivy (*Hedera helix*) is fidelity, and a daisy (*Bellis perennis*) represents innocence and simplicity. But never combine any "nice" flower with a foxglove (*Digitalis*) as it represents insincerity. So in a bouquet of love and well-meaning messages, it negates all of the positives." More jaws drop.

This secret floral code was created in England during the Victorian era and represents the high point of flowers as an expression of language. These collections of posies with specific meanings are called tussie-mussies and derive from nosegays, a small, hand-sized collection of flowers that was held up to one's nose to mute the aroma of open sewers in the cities of that period.

These Victorian-era arrangements are the 1800s floral version of text messages, as people used them to send clandestine signals to one another. While a red rose means passionate love, a yellow one represents friendship. A wrong color could send an unintentionally awkward message. During the heyday of tussie-mussies, young women would consult a variety of floral dictionaries to decipher the true meaning of a bouquet received from a suitor or friend.

Because I don't know what my clients will want to say using a floral cipher, I gather a wide variety of flora, some of which I clip from my yard and surrounding gardens. Even in February, there are evergreens as well as other plants that look attractive in a bouquet (see following box).

I show my clients how to arrange bouquets and instruct them to be watchful in the future of the message delivered by purchased flowers. I show the group pictures that I have taken of four different flower arrangements, each of which has a very different meaning. "This one, for instance, is for a hangover," I say. "The main flower is hens-and-chicks (*Sempervivum tectorum*), which means, welcome-home-husband-regardless-of-how-drunk-you-are." Norma muses that she should send that to her ex.

Boxwood (*Buxus*), which represents stoicism, is an adornment that quite a few are favoring, but I offer a warning before they commit it to their tussie-mussies. "Take a whiff," I suggest. When they start to smell the boxwood, their happy faces turn sour and the outcries are numerous:

"This is disgusting."

"God this is awful."

"What is this?!"

Helen finally identifies it and blurts out, "It smells like cat pee."

After this observation, the boxwood is shunned by the group. Many of the flowers that I bought from stores have little scent. "Why doesn't this rose smell like a rose?" asks Judy, placing her nose in the flower, puzzled over the lack of rose-familiar scent.

"It's because most flowers you buy in stores are bred to look nice and transport well rather than to have a strong fragrance," I say. "They won't smell like the roses in your garden or wild roses. If you want something that will kick off a lot of aroma, choose some of the herbs."

Some clients add rosemary and thyme to their bouquets to enhance their scent. Others struggle with the vocabulary of tussie-mussies and in the end decide to make a bouquet of what they believe most lovely.

A few of the crafted bouquets are too large, but with a bit of help and guidance they are scaled down to be more fitting for a hand to cradle. It takes experience to tie everything together so it will hold. Instead of grabbing many flowers and trying to tie the group together,

---

Arborvitae (*Thuja*)—Unchanging friendship

Baby's breath (*Gypsophila paniculata*)—Pure heart, festivity

Boxwood (*Buxus*)—Stoicism

Carnation (*Dianthus caryophyllus*) —Admiration

Carnation, deep red—Alas, for my poor heart

Carnation, pink –Woman's love, beauty, pride

Cedar (*Cedrus*)—Strength

Daffodil (*Narcissus*)—Respect, chivalry, gracefulness

Daisy (*Bellis perennis*) —Innocence, simplicity

Fern (*Tracheophyta*)—Fascination, sincerity

Forsythia (*Forsythia suspensa*)—Good nature

Holly (*Ilex aquifolium*)—Good will, domestic happiness

Ivy (*Hedera helix*)—Fidelity

Lily, tiger (*Lilium lancifolium*)—Wealth, pride

Moss (*Bryophyta*)—Maternal love

Periwinkle (*Vinca*)—Pleasures of memory

Primrose (*Primula vulgaris*)—Early youth

Rose (*Rosa*)—Love

Rose, red—I love you

Rose, yellow—Friendship

Rosemary (*Salvia rosmarinus*) —Remembrance

Sage (*Salvia officinalis*)—Virtue, wisdom, skill

Spruce (*Picea*)—Farewell, hope in adversity, immortality

Thyme (*Thymus vulgaris*)—Activity

it works better to layer in one or two at a time, wrapping each small bunch with florist wire. Experimenting, they soon create appropriately sized collections of plants. When finished, everyone has a nice bouquet that they are pleased with.

I create a small tussie-mussie for my wife, showing my clients that bigger is not necessarily better. I pick a red rose, two daffodils, a few sprigs of periwinkle, and a single primrose, which is roughly translated as "the graceful pleasures of young love." They think it is very beautiful, and when I bring it home to Juana, with a crib sheet of meanings, she thinks it equally lovely and sweet, rewarding me with a kiss on the cheek.

FEBRUARY CRAFT:
DISTILL HOMEMADE VANILLA EXTRACT

A tasty and simple craft for February is to make vanilla (Vanilla planifolia) extract. Once you create this, however, you may find it hard to go back to store-bought brands. You need just three things: Vanilla beans, vodka, and a small jar.

There are many types of vanilla beans: Madagascar, Tahitian, and Mexican are three of the most popular, each with its own specific flavor. You will need one bean for each ounce of vodka you use. Vanilla bean pods look much like green beans (Phaseolus vulgaris) from the outside, but they are very different on the inside. Inside each pod are very tiny seeds, difficult to see. It is the seeds, when mixed with alcohol, that create the extract.

To start, slice each bean vertically to expose the seeds. Many recipes place the sliced pod directly into the bottle with the seeds. I prefer to scrape the seeds out, cut up the pods, and place everything into the bottle. The dexterity and thought required for these extra steps creates a closer relationship between my clients and the vanilla. They also find soothing the vanilla fragrance that emanates during this preparation.

Next, pour one ounce of vodka into the bottle for every bean that is prepared. Any vodka will do. Making a colorful label with the date of creation finishes the exercise. Shake the bottle up once or twice a week and store it in a dark place; in two months a delicious vanilla extract will emerge.

FORSYTHIA AND PUSSY WILLOWS

Snow blankets my backyard and there is much to observe: tracks interspersed with countless shades and textures of bark and fallen branches. But hidden potential abounds, bringing a smile as an unexpected pleasure. In February, forcing forsythia and pussy willows (*Salix discolor*) is one such diversion. My mother loves both plants, as do many of the clients who attend the classes I teach at Meadow Ridge, a senior community in Redding, Connecticut. After they arrive to class, I show them a vase that I started a week earlier with pussy willows and forsythia that are now in full bloom.

"That's lovely. Are we going to get some?" asks June, an octogenarian with bright eyes who uses a walker for mobility. I nod. "It's simple to get this type of bloom," I start. "First, let's look for branches with big buds."

Earlier in the day, I had walked through foot-deep snow in my backyard to our row of forsythia. Shaking off its white overcoat, I had purposely cut a mix of stems, some that are fat with flower buds and those that do not have them. Pussy willows were easier to acquire at the local supermarket. I place the forsythia and pussy willows into two separate groups.

My clients examine the stems resting on the table. The forsythia appears gray to the eye, though there is a large visible difference between stems having fat and thin buds. Most of the clients are able to tell the difference and make their selections. One woman whose eyes are clouded with cataracts has a difficult time. She says little and appears frustrated, pulling back from the table where the stems sit.

"Emily, why don't you feel the buds with your hands? Here's one with fat buds. This other one has thin ones."

She nods and lets her thin, arthritic fingers glide over the stems. A smile brightens her face as she is now able to distinguish between the two types. Emily returns to the table to select the stems she will use for her bouquet.

I instruct the group to cut the stems with the pruners I brought and then to split the ends with a knife.

"Why do we have to split the stems?" asks Emily.

"It lets the branches absorb more water easily and will keep them alive longer," I reply. "They may even root for you in the vase if you change the water often enough."

More than half my clients, including Emily, need assistance splitting the stems but are patient as I make the rounds helping each one. After the stems are split, they wrap them in wet paper towels and place them into a small plastic bag. We repeat the exercise with the pussy willows.

"Put all the stems in warm water when you get back to your apartment and within a week you will get beautiful yellow forsythia flowers." Everyone smiles and prepares to go back to their rooms.

I always have extra material from my classes, so I gather a few leftovers to make a bouquet for my mother, who also lives at Meadow Ridge but did not attend today's class. She feels a bit under the weather, so I take the remaining stems and go to her apartment.

"This is such a nice surprise. Would you like a cup of tea?" she asks as I walk through her front door.

I accept her offer and ask for a vase so I can put her branches into it after we cut and slice them.

"I love pussy willows!" my mother exclaims. "Are those forsythia?"

My mother's face lights up and we find a vase that will hold the branches. She arranges them on her side table as we prepare the tea and set out a small plate of cookies. As we drink our tea, my mother chats with me while touching the soft, tiny pussy willow buds illuminated by the afternoon sun.

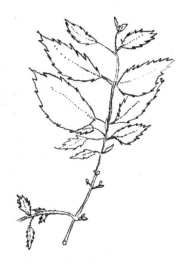

JACK AND THE BEANSTALK

I am often amazed at the creativity displayed by the children I mentor at the Children's Garden. Jack is perusing a pile of seed catalogs looking for interesting things to plant in the months to come. He perks up upon discovering uncommon types of beans: yin-yang, purple podded pole, and winged (*Psophocarpus tetragonolobus*). Jack wonders if we could plant these beans next month. I tell him that we can start them inside in March but perhaps we could also use the beans to create a story about him, Jack and the beanstalk.

"I hate that. Fairy tales are stupid."

"Why are you so upset Jack?"

"Because fairy tales are for babies and I am not a baby!"

"That's not true Jack. You said that you liked mythology from the Greeks and Romans; many fairy tales are not that different from classic mythology."

"I don't care. I don't want to make up a story for babies about giants and castles."

"You don't have to make up a story for babies. You can make up any story you like as long as it includes a boy named Jack and a beanstalk. It is limited only by your imagination. How about we work on it together?" Jack shrugs indifferently but says he will try. Jack finds it difficult to concentrate and is prone to violent flare ups. Working in the garden, however, is a calming influence on him, though care needs to be taken so that he does not become frustrated, have an outburst, and then potentially need to be restrained.

He starts to construct a story, picking out each word slowly and carefully. "As Jack looked in a seed catalog for ideas of what to plant in Spring he discovers . . ."

I then elaborate, ". . .when we get the beans in the mail, we discover that the seeds we receive are not the seeds we ordered. They look magical. They are striped with seven different colors and they glow in the dark. Jack is disappointed that the wrong beans were sent to us, but he's interested in the new ones and how they will grow."

Jack continues, "So Jack plants them in the garden. It usually takes beans a few days to grow from the soil, but when Mr. Keller and Jack visit the garden the next day, there is an eight-foot-high beanstalk with big, fat bean pods on the plant."

We continue for about fifteen minutes. The plant never stops bearing fruit, it has beautiful flowers that change color, and the beans taste like ice cream. With just a simple prompting, Jack is making up a wonderful, creative story. And soon our session is over, and it is time to leave the greenhouse where we are sitting in the sun and staying warm.

"This is great Jack, but we have to stop now and get you back to class."

"Okay, Mr. Keller. That was a lot of fun. Thanks."

"No problem. I think we should plant some beans soon for Summer."

"That'd be great. Especially if they glow in the dark."

LOL WITH YOUR INNER CHILD

Regardless of the client base, I believe that a successful horticultural-therapy session is always enhanced with humor and a few chuckles. Sometimes it can become more challenging when you have a roomful of clients at Ann's Place experiencing different stages of cancer; you don't want to say anything that will trigger a painful response. Humor must be used judiciously, elsewise it can backfire.

One of my techniques when I have an adult group is to reveal an unusual botanical historical fact, or to read something that they may not have heard of before that is germane to the session. If you ignite curiosity in an innocent and simple way, you will always win hearts. And sometimes get smiles. A class on forcing bulbs illustrates that point.

I thought that a poem on flowers would be a suitable way to start the day's exercise, but after reading through many, none really created the mood I was looking for. After reading William Wordsworth's "Daffodils" however, I remembered a Rocky and Bullwinkle cartoon from my youth that could do the trick. I brought my computer and a large display screen to augment my presentation.

"Now that we've finished with the mechanics of forcing bulbs, I think a poem would be nice," I say. I detect some discomfort and visual groans as I turn the computer toward my clients.

Bullwinkle prances over a field speaking the words "I wandered lonely as a cloud that floats on high o'er vales and hills, when all at once I saw a crowd, a host of golden daffodils; . . ." Clients start to smile, remembering their youth and the silliness of this cartoon. A few start laughing at the ungulate's rendition of an English classic they had heard years ago. When it is over they start talking among themselves about the cartoons of their youth and are ready to pot up some bulbs for early blooms and a link to Spring.

FEBRUARY OUTING: VISIT A GREENHOUSE

If you live in New England, February is a time when snow is often on the ground and your desire to experience Spring-like weather is high. No worries, as for most people there is a greenhouse within driving distance of your home. Walking through the doors, you are greeted with a rush of humid, oxygenated air that is fifty degrees warmer than you are used to. Here is a space full of life and growth.

These greenhouses come in a few flavors. For example, the NYBG's orchid show usually starts sometime in February. It is wondrous to see these rare and delicate plants inside a maze of spectacular greenhouses contrasted against piles of snow outside. Another type of greenhouse is used by commercial nurseries for plant propagation. Some will allow anyone to come in, tour their facilities, buy plants, and see row upon row of seedlings being grown for the season ahead. And then there are tiny greenhouses, like mine, that are unused, other than for storage, during the depth of Winter. Such small structures can be reviving on a cold, sunny day as they heat up quickly, allowing you to shed your outer layers to feel the warmth of the sun on your skin.

SENIOR SLIDES

Clients who reside in a nursing home, hospice, or similar facility often have a limited view of the outdoors. They have slight exposure to Nature save for a window or two at best. To compensate, before I start any class at Meadow Ridge, I put together a slideshow of what has been served up locally over the past few weeks. This might seem a futile exercise in February, but the Winter garden can be as interesting as a Spring or Summer one. For instance, this month my winterberry (*Ilex verticillata*) bushes are still filled with large red berries that create a wonderful contrast against the snow.

But just hours before my class, a flock of robins visited my yard and within ten minutes removed every berry from the bushes. I was fortunate to be at the window with camera in hand to record this feeding. The only berries left are a few on the ground that the robins dislodged but missed consuming. I show my clients a picture of the bushes with a full load of berries, one of the robins eating them, and then a final one of the berry-free bushes. Seeing that display, my clients start to ask questions.

"Are there really robins this time of year?"

"Will other birds eat the berries?"

"Why weren't the berries eaten earlier in the season?"

With each question comes a discussion of Winter and the interdependence of animals and plants. I then ask, "So did any of you see similar things at your homes?" Sylvia remembers a crabapple (*Malus*) tree at her mother's house that used to be visited by birds in Fall. Another remembers that she used to have a northern bayberry (*Myrica pensylvanica*) bush nearby her home filled with tiny and fragrant gray berries in Winter.

"Do birds eat bayberries?" Sylvia asks. I tell her that warblers, in particular, like bayberries. All the trees and bushes, like the winterberry near my house, attract different birds at different times. The crabapple's tiny, shriveled fruits are typically the last to be eaten before Spring.

I also have photos of birds on my feeders, so my clients get to see woodpeckers, bluebirds, cardinals, pine siskins, sparrows, and other birds that are wintering in my yard. Other images show leafless trees casting long shadows on the snow, creating a pattern that does not exist during the warmer months.

These images foster an attention that was not there when we started the class. Senior clients in these living situations are often placed in front of a television set and pay little attention to the drone of a movie or game show. But now they are engaged, attempting to remember trees and plants from their past that have meaning and— more important—a memory that they can retrieve.

"Is the snow now good for sledding?"

"I had a white birch (*Betula papyrifera*) in my yard."

"Why do some birds remain and others fly south?"

Each image creates a launching point for discussions with my clients, remembering loved ones and homes that exist only as a fading memory. Soon we will start our exercise. But for now they are engaged with the season at hand as well as those in their memories.

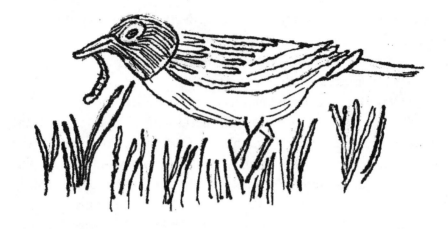

GARDENING HEAD CASES

"It's hard to make the glasses fit. You have quite a big head."

Silence. (Oops.) Then laughter.

Let me start from the beginning.

There are a few snowdrops (*Galanthus nivalis*) and crocuses (*Crocus vernus*) that have sprouted, but everything else is dormant. After all, it is February and we are in New England. But there is still the opportunity to plant things this time of year. Grassheads, a homemade version of a Chia pet, is a favorite Winter activity. The first time I tried it, I was unsure how well it would be received; it turns out silly crafts go over well with my clients.

After everyone arrives to class and settles in, I turn away, removing my glasses and replacing them with a pair of novelty Groucho Marx ones, complete with nose and mustache. As they all stare at me, I pass out identical pairs to everyone. "You need to wear these glasses to get into the proper mood and gain inspiration," I say. "Look across the table at your friends for grasshead models if you don't have a good idea of what type you want to make." Everyone struggles with their Groucho glasses, but soon the table is encircled with silly-looking clients. Giggles and smiles emerge. I bring out three sample grassheads that were made by Juana, Charlotte, and me. Charlotte's is the most interesting of the three as it expresses a post-impressionist, Cubist design with eyes and facial features askew. I then demonstrate how to make one.

It's quite simple. A stocking, some grass seed, soil, a few rubber bands, fake eyes, pom-poms, pipe cleaners, felt, glue gun, and you have everything you need. I tell my clients that they can make as many as they desire; everyone creates a set of twins.

"To start, put a footsie stocking inside a small bowl or pint glass and stretch the opening over the lip, so layers of ryegrass (*Lolium multiflorum*) seed and soil can be placed inside. Be careful about where you place the grass seed, as badly sowed seeds can sprout faux hair in all the wrong spots," I say.

"How do these look?" asks Sabrina.

"They're perfect. You gave it angry eyes. Anyone we know?" I reply.

Another client uses felt to create eyebrows. She sprinkles grass seeds around the ears she forms with rubber bands so an infrequently barbered old-man look is effected. The ladies start laughing as they comment that many of their husbands are an inspiration for their placement (or lack thereof) of seed hair.

Each head emerges with a different personality and style. There is an undercurrent of chatter and observations while everyone is concentrating on their heads to create unique looks. By the end of the class, everyone is proud of their creations. I give each client a small paper cup where the grasshead will sit, wicking up water for the seeds.The silly exercise works; it is now time for a group picture.

At the next class a few clients return with fuzzy heads.

"I love this," says Mavis. "This is so cute."

"There is too much hair here," says Leena, who also brought in her grasshead. "But I can always trim."

SHOVELING SNOW, SOWING SEEDS

The warming rays of the sun turn a blind eye to the snow surrounding our house, timidly bouncing off rather than being absorbed. There is still a foot of white in our backyard, while in town down the hill, barely a pile of snow can be found.

The greenhouse and the cold frames—boxes with transparent covers that act as passive solar-energy reservoirs—have been shoveled after each snowfall so they would not collapse. Mounds of snow still surround them. With a warm sun beating down, Charlotte and I go outside. She carries an ice chipper and I a shovel. Our aim is to dig out the areas around the greenhouse and make it less dangerous to walk and work around the garden. Charlotte's interest, however, is more focused on climbing the piles of snow and licking the tiny balls of ice that stick to her mittens.

After removing much of the accumulated snow, I carefully pull away icy sheets from our herb garden with the hope that some of the perennials will reemerge in the weeks to come so we can retire some of our store-bought McCormick spices. Charlotte peers with interest into the newly revealed beds.

While most of my vegetable garden is cold and covered by a reflective sheen, the cold frame and hoop houses are toasty. A waft of warm, moist air and the smell of rotting vegetation greet me as I lift one of the cold-frame panels. Charlotte looks for things to nibble on, removing her mittens so she can better grab any remaining greens.

The Swiss chard (*Beta vulgaris* subsp. *vulgaris*), romaine (*Lactuca sativa* var. *longifolia*), and mizuna (*Brassica juncea* var. *japonica*) greens are no more. I pull their shriveled and rotting leaf remnants from the garden and drop them onto a nearby compost heap covered with snow. The soil, warm to the touch, gives them up easily and weeds have started to sprout.

But a few greens have wintered over. The winter marvel lettuce (*Lactuca sativa*) is perky with a small head about three inches in diameter. I remove a tiny leaf and enjoy its sweet taste and crisp texture. Charlotte also samples the tender leaves and wants more. She happily stuffs two more leaves into her mouth. I am hoping that the warmth and Spring light will accelerate its growth so the lettuce will be ready for harvest in the next month. Charlotte then grabs my trowel and pushes it down into the soil nearly six inches.

It is early, but having nothing to lose save a few seeds, we decide to sow a few early Spring plants. After working some compost into the soil, we etch a few rows to plant different greens and radishes (*Raphanus sativus*). Charlotte is not as disciplined as I, so the rows and spacing of seeds are less defined; but it matters little as any growth would be a small miracle right now. With luck, and warmer weather, we may see some sprouts in a week or so.

The rest of the yard struggles to show signs of growth. Walking around the perimeter of the house with me, Charlotte spots a clump of recently sprouted snowdrops. She picks a few for her mother and grandmother. We both hope that this is a good sign that Winter is about to turn.

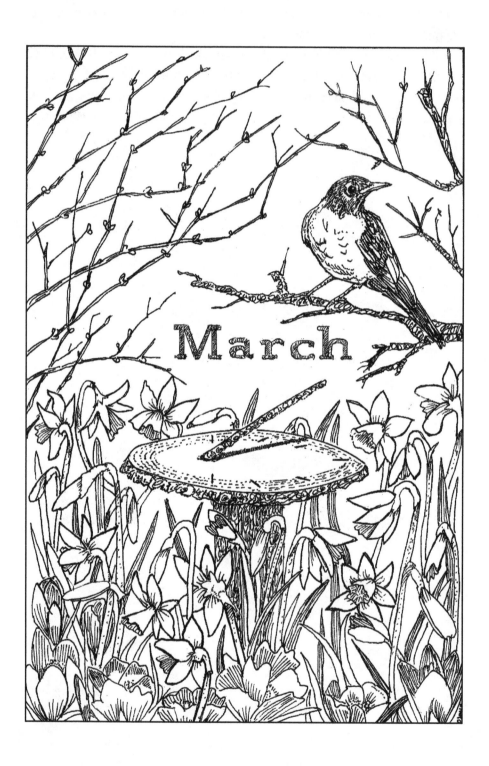

MARCH: A FICKLE MONTH

The old saying that March comes in like a lion and out like a lamb is an inaccurate Nature proverb. Sometimes March comes in like a lamb and out like a lion, as a mild Winter gives way to a cold, delayed Spring. It is a month of confusion and frustration as the daylight lengthens, leading to the Spring equinox and the anticipation of warmer days and nights.

Flexibility and patience is needed this month more than any other, as the melting snow can be refreshed many times. The return of certain birds to feeders as well as the emergence of early bulbs popping out of the thawing soil herald warmer days to come.

A LONE CLIENT

Attendance varies greatly for my classes at Ann's Place because my clients are coping with cancer. Today, eleven people signed up for my class on how to make a sachet. Class is about to start and I am by myself in the art room. Total no-show. Ten minutes into class time, I start to put everything away, readying myself to go home. As I turn toward the door, a diminutive woman approaches me.

"I'm not sure if this is the right time," she says, embarrassed. "I get very confused nowadays with the chemo treatments I've been getting." She looks around and sees that no one else is here. Her eyes start to water.

"I was really looking forward to this. Perhaps I should call my husband to pick me up," she says, turning to leave.

I tell her to stay and that we can have a session between the two of us. She doesn't want to put me to any trouble, but I say that since we are both here we should just go on. A little smile turns up on her face. Removing her coat reveals a very thin and pale frame to match a face distinguished by high cheekbones and deeply sunken blue eyes.

"What is your name?" I ask.

"Delores."

"Delores, what is your favorite scent?"

"Lavender *(Lavandula angustifolia)*. It reminds me of when I was young."

I add that my mother's favorite scent is lilac *(Syringa vulgaris)* because her mother grew lilac bushes in her backyard. Delores smiles and agrees that it is a wonderful smell. I tell her that one of my favorite smells is that of pickles—flavored with dill (*Anethum graveolens*), bay leaves (*Laurus nobilis*), and vinegar—as it reminds me of when I used to eat lunch with my father outside in Summer. Delores begins to relax. With that I begin our session.

"One thing to decide when making a sachet is how and where it will be used. For example, if you wanted to create a sachet for the kitchen or bathroom, it would probably have a very different scent than one for a drawer where you keep your fine scarfs." Delores nods, taking notes on a pad she pulls out of her purse.

"First consider how to combine different scents. You have to be careful, because certain combinations sit better than others. I've brought twelve essential and seven fragrant oils, plus several herbs and spices. All their scents fall into four categories: sweet, sour, vegetable, and animal." I then describe each one and suggest that she choose a fundamental base scent and then surround it with related ones.

"Well I think I will pick nutmeg (*Myristica fragrans*)," she says after sniffing different oils, spices, and herbs. To unlock the nutmeg's scent, she starts to grind it with a pestle. "Oh my," she says after a few strokes release the nutmeg's essence. She says that her chemotherapy has made her unable to discern most scents. Nutmeg is one of the few that she still perceives. She then looks over the other options and chooses cinnamon (*Cinnamomum verum*), some chamomile (*Matricaria chamomilla*), and touches of a few other spices.

She marvels at the changing complexity and complementary nature of her selections as they combine in her bowl; new scents are released with each turn of the spoon. Crushing the cinnamon with a mortar and pestle releases even more aromas. A different story and memory of her past emerge with each inhalation, creating conversation. Delores is satisfied with her mix but now we need to add an essential oil to her selections.

"How about peppermint (*Mentha piperita*)?" I suggest. "It's very complementary to what you have put together, and it will bind well with the oak moss that we need to use as a fixative. We'll place it in a separate bowl so you can smell it by itself." When making a sachet, either oak moss or cellulose fiber acts as a medium to absorb and slowly release scents.

She agrees. (Peppermint can help minimize nausea, a byproduct of chemotherapy.) After mixing the oak moss with peppermint and adding it to her selections, she inhales deeply. "This is incredible. It's nothing like I thought it would be. Thank you." I smile, telling Delores that I don't like to give canned recipes to clients and prefer to let them explore and discover their own blends.

More stories and memories emerge while she decorates her sachet bag with colorful Sharpie markers and stuffs her mixture into it. And before I know it, Delores is waving goodbye, happy, with sachet in hand.

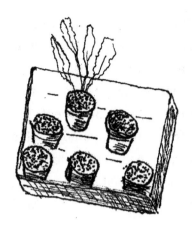 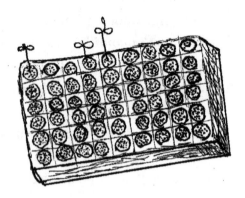

BABY STEPS

With morning temperatures well below freezing and my storage shed encased in snow, it appears foolish to start up seedlings. Yet with only a few weeks before Spring and the emergence of early garden growth, I know that I need to start up the flats of flowers, greens, and herbs that will adorn our grounds during Summer and Fall. Donning coats, gloves, and boots, Charlotte and I make our way out to the shed, me crunching through a foot-plus of half-melted snow covered by a crust of ice, and she shimmering as would a fairy over a magical field of frosting.

The doors to the shed are blocked with packed snow. After we pull away the frozen impediment and pry one door open, we enter to retrieve a pair of grow-light stands as well as the plywood platform that holds my seedling trays. The mouse bait along the walls is half gone, indicating that a few rodents have used the shed as Winter residence. I will discover their shriveled bodies in Spring when I clean it out.

Other needed supplies sit in the greenhouse on the other side of my yard. Making our way and opening the door, Charlotte and I are greeted by a blast of eighty-degree air, a happy contrast to the freezing temperature outside and the dark shed we just left. "Pampi, it's hot in here," she says, removing her snow jacket. I pick her up, placing her on a shelf as I start selecting the seeding trays that we will need later in the day. Charlotte motions for me to remove her snow pants, but I tell her they need to stay on. The slight perfume of manure scents the greenhouse, and I notice a few heart-shaped leaves of wood sorrel (*Oxalis acetosella*) germinating in an old flower pot I didn't remove last Fall. A small leak in the skylight has kept it watered. Charlotte happily eats the leaves I give her.

I collect the seed trays and tell Charlotte that it is time to go in. She wants to stay warm in the greenhouse, but I lure her with the prospect of fresh bread later and she relents. After we close the door on the greenhouse, I lift her over the fence and let her slide down a steep pile of shoveled snow into the driveway where Juana is waiting with open arms.

We set up our potting area in the kitchen, where the soil that I had brought in the day before has warmed to room temperature. Unlike potting up bulbs, we need to spread the soil over the seed trays into ice-cube sized cells. Charlotte does well with this activity, as she picks up chunks of soil and spreads them over the trays with a spoon. She tries to fill every hole with soil, and I compliment her on a good job. She looks up, smiles, and continues preparing the trays, humming to herself. Soon it is time to plant.

Charlotte helps me plant the larger Swiss chard (*Beta vulgaris* subsp. *vulgaris*) and spinach (*Spinacia oleracea*) seeds as her little fingers can pick them up individually and deftly put them into a cell of soil. She starts out placing three seeds per cell then starts to improvise and drops more into the cells after an initial planting. Those cells will need much thinning in a month.

I use a dial seed sower to distribute the tiny seeds of greens as my stubby fingers are unable to neatly plant them into the individual cells. Working together we encourage each other on the progress the other makes. Soon we have all the seeds in soil and ready to place on the heating mats underneath the grow lights. Within a few days, they start to germinate. Charlotte is pleased at the growth. "Pampi, when will we be able to eat them?" she asks. I tell her in a month we will be able to sample some greens. She smiles and then takes my hand, leading us to our next adventure.

MARCH CRAFT: REGROW FOOD FROM SCRAPS

Though it is too early to start anything outside in the garden unless you have a cold frame, you can regrow vegetables now from scraps that you would normally throw out. It is a simple exercise that you can do with many different plants.

The key to this vegetable-growing shortcut is to slice and save the growing part of the plant you are using. For example, the bottoms of celery (Apium graveolens), cabbage (Brassica oleracea var. capitata), scallions (Allium fistulosum), and romaine lettuce (Lactuca sativa var. longifolia), to mention a few, should be saved after consuming the upper parts of the plant. If you leave a few inches intact on the bottoms and put them in water, which should be changed every day, within a week you will get new growth and yummy greens to eat. The same can be done with the tops of carrots (Daucus carota var. sativus), which will sprout new decorative and edible greens. You can use this technique for many other foods, but these five give a quick return of growth in the waning days of Winter.

GROWING UP

Many of the baker's dozen of clients who arrive today at Ann's Place confide that they don't know what to expect, but the prospect of a Spring garden in early March is enough to fill the room.

"While many of you may think it too early to start a garden, I have to tell you that I've been late in starting my greens for early Spring planting. If you have a window that gets a good amount of light during the day, you can start a garden today in a window box or flat that should start giving you enough greens for a simple salad by mid to late April. In fact, some of the radish (*Raphanus sativus*) seeds I've picked out for you today mature in less than one month." This piques the interest of the group and starts an ad hoc discussion.

"How deep should I plant the seeds?" asks Lucy. "Great question. It's a function of the size of the seed. Tiny seeds like lettuce should be covered with an eighth to a quarter inch of soil, while larger ones like squash can go as deep as one inch. The reason for this is that a seed has only so much stored energy before it needs to tap the nutrients in the soil and light. If you plant a small seed too deep, the sprout may die out because it exhausts all the energy in the seed before its leaves can tap the power of the sun for photosynthesis."

"Can we plant peppers and tomatoes now?" asks Heather. "Not for what we're doing. Those plants require higher temperatures and more light than you get at this time of year. It'll be at least another month before you want to start tomatoes."

"When can we place our boxes outside?" inquires Rosa. "It depends. If we have nice sunny days when the temperatures get into the low fifties, it's a good idea to put the box outside for as long as it's warm, and then bring the box back in when it cools down in the evening. It won't be until late March or early April when you can leave these boxes outside all the time."

After we clear the air of questions, I then reveal some of the tricks of planting seeds.

"How do you think you should plant some of these seeds?" I ask as I pass around two different packets of seeds—red leaf (*Lactuca sativa*) and miners lettuce (*Claytonia perfoliata*)—both of which are very tiny. As my clients strain to see the seeds, I sense that doubts are creeping into their minds as to how easy the task will prove to be. I then offer a hand seed sower to each of them that will make the chore a snap. The class exhales a collective sigh of relief after I tell them how to use this tool. It is time to prepare the soil.

We need to wet and mix the soil before planting, because if you don't, the seeds will float around as the mixture attempts to absorb the water. I always find that clients vary between mud lovers who will mix the soil, manure, and water with bare hands and those who will only work with gloves and a trowel. People pair off to prepare their soil.

"What is the right way to plant?" asks Jane, expressing the worry of the others.

"There is no right or wrong way. You can either create rows or broadcast seeds randomly." I then bring out two different seed flats that I had started a few weeks back. One looks like a lawn of greens; the other has neat rows like a farmer's field.

"Is that what we will get in a few weeks?" asks Jane. I nod yes.

And with that the group starts to sow their Spring greens with the hope that they will be able to fill their plates with a home-grown salad in the weeks to come.

SCHOOL'S IN

Typically the fifth season in New England—mud season—starts around now when the top layer of soil melts slightly, creating an organic ooze with gelatin-like consistency. This mire often causes an unanticipated tumble, or it collects more deeply into a quicksand-like quagmire that swallows a boot with a quick gulp. But this year is atypical. We have had a nearly perfect melt in the Northeast with Goldilocks-like weather so that the soil is moist yet can be walked on and worked. Given these conditions I am hopeful that I can work with the children at Green Chimneys to plant radishes and peas (*Pisum sativum*) in the garden.

I walked out to the Children's Garden a few days ago, lifted up the Agribon covers on the hoop houses, and saw that the cauliflower (*Brassica oleracea* var. *botrytis*), mustard greens (*Brassica juncea*), and some of the lettuces were coming back from a rough Winter. The carrots were intact. I pulled one from the soil for sampling; it had a distinctive snap upon biting, and was sweet and ready to eat. Kale (*Brassica oleracea* var. *sabellica*) had sprouted in an adjacent row, sending up baby leaves that can be harvested within a few weeks.

Any garden on the cusp of Spring will let you know how well you dealt with the weeds of the prior year. If you did a good job in Fall, your rows will be fallow and empty. A poor job will cause your rows to be filled with more weeds than you care to count. Some plants, like dill and fennel (*Foeniculum vulgare*), go from desired herb to invasive weed as their seed pods and roots generously spread their progeny.

But my desire to explore the garden today is dampened. It is a raw rainy day and the children are wary to work outside.

"Let's plan the garden for Spring rather than go out in the rain," I tell my students, giving each a pencil, paper, and a few seed catalogs. "Look at the catalogs and first write down a list of what you want to plant and then draw a picture of where your choices should be placed in the garden."

The students look at the catalogs and start to ask questions.

"Can we plant watermelons now?"

"I like oranges, can we plant the seeds?"

"When will the flowers bloom?"

A simple review of seed catalogs is opening their eyes to the potential that can be realized in the garden in just a few months. Gershon spends more than fifteen minutes carefully examining a Parks Seed catalog, amazed at the different flowers and vegetables he finds. "I didn't think peas had so many pretty flowers," he observes.

They then start to draw their garden pictures and are pleased with their progress, even though the chill and rain outside has thwarted their day in the garden. Such references help us define the season and the chores to come. It is hard to imagine that just a week ago the only grasses discernible were sparse patches covered with snow mold. But now it is time to get ready for early Spring planting.

MARCH OUTING: FIND FOOD

Soil is still unworkable in many places, but tasty snacks can be found outside in the first growth of March. What many of us would call weeds, early settlers and indigenous Americans would call fresh vegetables, which would be particularly welcome at the end of a long Winter. One of the easiest, and most pervasive, greens to collect in New England is garlic mustard (Alliaria petiolata), which was first spotted on Long Island, New York, in 1868. Having both medicinal and food properties, the early shoots of garlic mustard are good in a salad as a tasty, tart leaf.

Early violets (Viola sororia) can also be munched on, as well as sheep sorrel (Rumex acetosella), which becomes rather large and too tart to consider in another month or two, depending upon the weather. Wild garlic, or ramsons (Allium ursinum), and onions (Allium canadense) are tasty accompaniments to salads and can be added to pasta dishes for an added kick. And there is the ubiquitous dandelion (Taraxacum officinale) that can always be found under the melting snow.

CELEBRATING THE SUN

A favorite client activity around the Spring equinox is to build sundials on wood slabs. As clients arrive to class, they can spot a few of the eleven thousand daffodils (*Narcissus*) unveiling themselves in the back of Ann's Place. Grape hyacinths (*Muscari armeniacum*) are emerging along a stone-dust path, their spears of tiny grape-like purple blooms poking through the soil among the greening tall fescue (*Festuca arundinacea*).

"This is what all of you will be creating today, a sundial," I say, showing them a sample. "My wife, who is vastly more talented than I, made this one and it is accurate to our longitude and latitude." Adjacent to the art room where we are having our class is a concrete-block retaining wall. We all leave the classroom so I can place Juana's sundial on it, adjusting it to tell the proper time, and my clients can see the shadow of the dial indicating the current standard time.

They are now looking more interested, so I continue after we reenter the building. "It is guaranteed that nearly any sundial you purchase will be inaccurate, as it needs to be timed, so to speak, to the latitude and longitude where it will reside. For people in the New York City area . . ." I then describe the mathematics of sundials and how they work. While the class is somewhat interested in sundial theory, it is clear they want to start building their own.

Unlike other activities we do, building a sundial requires more rigor as there are two important things to consider. The first is transferring hour lines to the correct position on the dial face. The other is to set the gnomon, which casts the shadow on the dial, on a specific center line of the dial aligned with high noon.

In keeping with a horticultural-therapy theme, I cut the dials from black locust (*Robinia pseudoacacia*) and black birch (*Betula lenta*) trees that fell on my property during the year. The gnomons are cut from Japanese maple (*Acer palmatum*), sugar maple (*Acer saccharum*), black birch, and oak (*Quercus*). I cut the disks to a uniform thickness and then use my chop saw to cut each gnomon so that it will lay on the dial at an angle of forty-one degrees, which is the latitude of the New York City metropolitan area. Given these materials, a series of instructions, and templates, the group sets off to work.

The typical casual chatter is deferred for quiet determination as each client focuses on drawing their lines on the dials accurately. "Remember, nothing is wrong until you commit a permanent marker to the wood, and even then, we can sand most anything off," I advise.

Sherrie becomes frustrated early on as she is having a hard time stenciling the sundial hour lines on her dial using transfer paper. "Nothing is wrong with what you are doing," I assure her. "Just determine which direction you want your sundial to point toward and put down the template like this." I demonstrate how to transfer the information and she relaxes. A slight smile emerges.

"The fun part of this is how you personalize the sundial and what type of designs you decide upon. Do your designs freehand, without transfer paper," I tell the group.

As the session continues, everyone becomes more comfortable with the task and starts to create different and unique designs. Chatter starts slowly and soon people are talking and sharing ideas as has been typical with other sessions. Some start to ask questions about sundials:

"Could I give this to my mother in Arizona?" (Yes, but it would be very inaccurate, because the latitude and longitude are different there.)

"What does a sundial look like on the North Pole?" (A gnomon that is straight up with a dial having twenty-four equally spaced hour slashes.)

"How will we attach the stick to the dial?" (It's a secret that I will demonstrate to everyone later.)

Soon each client has a sundial that will accurately tell time in their backyard. All are very happy with their accomplishment.

"I never would have thought about doing something like this," says Jamal. "It turned out better than I ever could have imagined."

After the clients finish their pieces, I spray them a few times with a quick-drying lacquer to hold up against the elements. "You should consider putting at least three coats of spar varnish on these if you want them to last outside," I suggest.

I then tell them how to set their sundials at night using the reference of the North Star, or during the day with a compass, giving them an instruction sheet to help them remember the process. Cleaning up, I notice that the sun is still visible in the sky, and with a glance, see that Juana's sundial sitting on the wall outside is still telling time accurately.

CHARLOTTE SALADS

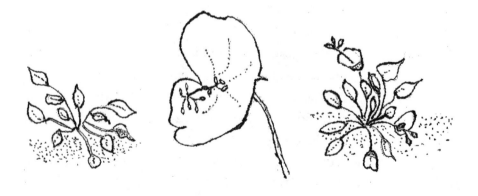

Charlotte has Spring fever and doesn't want to stay inside. She is itching to sample the outdoors. For her, that still means putting nearly everything in her mouth, ranging from small rocks to large sticks. But I figure it is time to get her into the garden, to show her what we can put in her mouth from the garden at this time of year.

Some greens have over-wintered nicely. The spinach I planted last September is pushing out some shoots as well as the bok choy (*Brassica rapa* subsp. *chinensis*). The best crops are the heart-shaped miners lettuce and corn salad (*Valerianella locusta*). They are a tasty snack and very sweet this time of year. We have a surfeit of crunchy little leaves that are ideal for Charlotte's small and mostly toothless mouth. My raised beds are the perfect height for her to grab and play with the soil. She digs in, moving her hands in circles across the black, warming earth. She wants a little snack so I feed her leaf after leaf that she sucks down using her tiny pink tongue.

The garden is a new experience for her and she can't decide how to react. What should she put in her mouth versus what should she just grab? Sometimes I think it is too much for her to handle. I often consider what she will remember of her grandfather and his love for gardening. Regardless, Spring is here and I will just keep feeding Charlotte from the garden, letting her get well within reach of the lettuce but blocking her sight from the foxglove (*Digitalis*) that has established itself. You can never be too careful with those you love.

NEW CHILDREN

The cold of Winter is but a memory with only a few piles of dirty snow remaining in the back of parking lots. Like my yard, the Children's Garden at Green Chimneys has thawed, and the hoop houses are giving us an early start with many of the rows ready for sowing as the soil is warm underneath their Agribon covers.

Last week all the carrots were harvested from one of the raised beds. The turnip greens (*Brassica rapa* subsp. *rapa*) I had planted in

Fall are resprouting in another row and will be ready for harvest in the next month. A row of spinach that we had planted as a lark last September wintered over nicely, now sporting four-inch rosettes. The leaves are exceptionally sweet.

The academic quarters have changed, and I am greeted by a new group of students. All of them are excited to be in the garden. I task my first charge, Linda, to clean up our herb garden and dress it up with Sweet Peet, an organic mulch. I give Linda a pair of garden pruners and we start to remove old stalks of mint (*Mentha*).

I ask her if she can identify the herb we are pruning. She can't.

"Rub your hands on the stalks and see if you can guess," I say. She removes her gloves and rubs the stalks against her two hands and moves them to her nose. At first she looks puzzled but then she grins saying, "It's mint, isn't it?"

I have her do the same to the herbs that we were not cutting, including some creeping thyme (*Thymus serpyllum*), oregano (*Origanum vulgare*), and lavender. The fresh scent of the herbs is refreshing her as she tires from our morning chores. When she starts to become bored or finds difficulty with a task, I take her back to the herb garden for a quick aromatherapy break, and I ask her what each herb reminds her of. Lavender reminds her of perfume. "This smells like pizza," she says of the oregano.

After I return Linda to class, I work with a group of children to prepare one of the garden rows for planting. To prep the soil, we need to add compost. Our pile of compost, which is a combination of manure from the barns, old hay, and food scrap wastes from the Green Chimney's kitchen, is over ten feet high and much of it is still frozen. I instruct Ben to work around the edges lower on the pile and in the sun rather than dig into the shaded middle. He does not listen and strikes the side of the pile at shoulder-height ineffectively. He becomes frustrated and throws his shovel at the pile. He walks away.

"Ben, if you go with your shovel around the lower sides and top where it is sunny, it will be much easier," I say. "You can become king of the mountain. Let me show you."

I pick up his shovel, climb to the top of the pile and start to scrape off the warm compost. Ben looks on and asks, "How did you know that the top would be melted?"

"Ben, this pile was rock solid only a few weeks ago, but since then the sun has been warming it up so parts have started to melt. It takes a long time, however, for the sun and warmth to reach the middle of the pile, which is why it is still too hard to shovel where you were before. By removing the top and lower sides of the pile, we are helping the sun melt it faster."

Ben seems to understand, scampering up to the top of the pile and throwing shovels of compost into the wheelbarrow below. Pushing the shovel's blade deep into the compost, he fills up the wheelbarrow a half a dozen times. He is happy to be working up a sweat and getting the beds ready for planting.

I take my next charge, Eric, to the cold frame near the greenhouse to collect the lettuce seedlings that are hardening off after we started them last month in the greenhouse. Our cold frames are both thrifty and clever. We use rotting bales of hay to form a sheltered space, and old storm windows are placed on top to capture the sun during the day. At the end of the day we lay down discarded horse blankets over them to hold the heat. These structures are more accurately called warm frames, as the rotting hay creates heat via an exothermic reaction. This morning it was thirty-seven degrees outside, yet the warm frame was emitting puffs of humid air from its sides.

As we remove the storm windows, I have Eric place his hand within the first layer of hay. "That's really hot," he says pulling his fingers out. I then explain to him that the decaying hay is generating heat, which in turn keeps our seedlings warm. He thought it was cool that old hay would heat our plants.

In looking over our stock, we have a good selection of vegetables to choose from: broccoli (*Brassica oleracea* var. *italica*), lettuce, arugula (*Eruca vesicaria* subsp. *sativa*), cauliflower, and spinach. I grab a flat and a half of romaine lettuce, place the cell packs in the wagon and start to walk with Eric back to the garden.

Though the wagon is weighted down, Eric keeps pulling hard. On a few occasions he wants me to pull it, and I tell him I will help him, but not do his job for him. He understands and we share in the task.

Eric and Fred, my next student, will spend the rest of their time planting lettuce. It takes dexterity to separate the seedlings from the cell packs, but after a few simple demonstrations, each is able to remove the root balls intact. Both students keenly observe how the intertwined roots hold the soil in the rectangular shape of each cell. Thin white roots contrasting against the dark soil create an interesting pattern unique to each seedling. On the rare occasions when the soil falls apart, each believes that they have ruined or killed the plant.

"I killed it! I can't do anything right," says Fred who starts to sob. "It's okay Fred," I reply, placing an assuring hand on his shoulder. "For some reason the roots didn't hold on to the soil, but the plant is fine and the roots strong. We just need to be careful in planting it. Let me show you." We tenderly place it into a hole we dig; Fred smooths the soil around it and it stands up like the others. He starts to calm down and offers up a slight grin.

When working with children who are planting seedlings, one of the best ways to teach is to work as a team, switching jobs and letting the student take the lead. Both Eric and Fred, however, like to remove the seedlings from the cell pack and plant them, leaving me to dig the holes.

The children are beginning to get used to working in the garden regardless of weather. When they visit, all hope for a veggie snack, but this time of year the pickings are slim. The sorrel (*Rumex acetosa*) is just beginning to come up though the spinach is nearly full sized. I give each child a morsel of spinach, telling them to be patient as more vegetables will be forthcoming. They nod with approval while munching the meager harvest our garden has to offer in March.

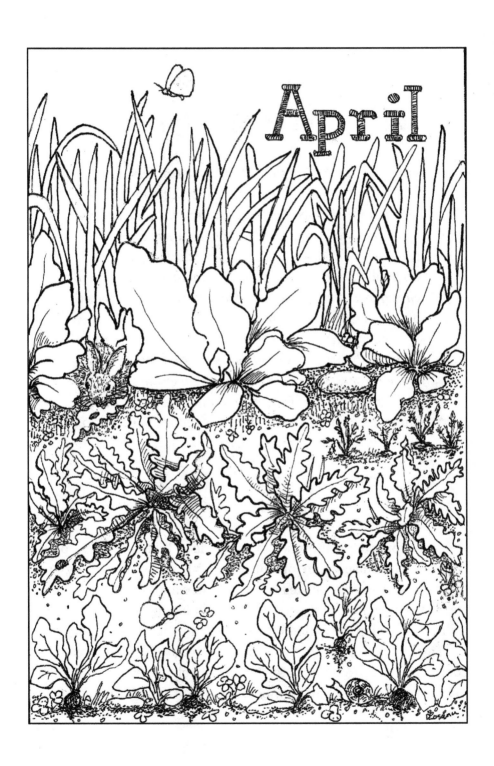

APRIL: STARTING TO GROW

Even during the harshest April, most plants come to life. Some arrive and depart in a blink, while others thrive until the deep chills of Autumn. Bulbs are the most likely to be confused by the weather, as crocuses (Crocus), daffodils (Narcissus), hyacinths (Hyacinthus orientalis), and tulips (Tulipa) sometimes make their emergence, simultaneously, if a cold period is followed by an excessively long warm spell.

The ground morphs from a dingy gray and brown to a lively green. Countless flies and bugs hatch, looking for food to consume and flowers to pollinate. The persistent cold is over and an undulating, gentle, and embracing warmth makes us realize that there is no turning back: Spring is here.

FIRST WALKS

It is a cool but sunny afternoon at Ann's Place. Clients bundle up with scarfs, gloves, and coats to join me in a walk to see what is emerging in the garden. A few are unsteady on their feet and need help walking. Ready to enjoy the afternoon, we exit the building and stand next to a railing overseeing the daffodils below in a drainage area.

This patch has over seven thousand bulbs planted, creating a complex pattern to appreciate. A river of yellow, cream, white, and orange flowers waving in the wind, the colorful daffodils dominate the view.

"From up high," I tell clients, "you can see the daffodils almost like cloud formations. Does anyone see a pattern or something besides flowers?"

"I see a bench."

"Is there a bird there?"

"How about a snake?"

With that simple suggestion, clients start speaking among themselves, trading stories about how their gardens grow in Spring. We move on to the mint (*Mentha*) walk and herb garden.

Though there is not much to sample now, some of the early mints are emerging as well as the sorrel (*Rumex acetosa*) and chives (*Allium schoenoprasum*). I give everyone a taste of the sorrel and tell them to rub the emerging mints. The fresh tastes and scents roll over them, and smiles come to their faces with this early harvest.

Everyone is surprised by the plethora of tree and bush buds that are swollen, ready to burst. Tiny slivers of red, blue, pink, green, and white strain to embrace the sun. "Here is a plant you want to avoid," I point out. I cut a branch of Japanese barberry (*Berberis thunbergii*) from a bush that has lodged itself in the rocks. I hold up the stem, revealing to the class the orange innards as well as its spiky stems. "If you have this in your yard, you want to get rid of it. It may be pretty but it will take over," I say, and then point to the wetlands area beyond the fence that protects the gardens from the local deer herds. It is filled with Japanese barberry bushes, which are choking out most of the undergrowth. Skunk cabbages (*Symplocarpus foetidus*) are attempting to leaf out and flower, but the blanket of greening barberry hinders their progress.

We appreciate the lack of background noise, as landscapers have yet to descend en masse to clean nearby properties. Houses are easily spotted through a skeletal screen of deciduous tree trunks and limbs, as the leaf canopy in the adjoining wetlands has yet to fill in. Dried seed pods on the Virginia ryegrass (*Elymus virginicus*) flutter in the light breeze that follows us on our walk.

Garlic mustard (*Alliaria petiolata*) is emerging out of the leaf litter. "Here is something else you want to avoid," I say pointing to an attractive green floret. I attempt to pull it out but it snaps off at the stem. "This is not what you want to do when you try to get rid of garlic mustard," I mutter, somewhat defeated. "Pretty soon we will have to start weeding in earnest." I pull off leaflets offering them to my students to sample; they are pungent with the scent of garlic. Most try my offering, though they are divided as to its suitability in a salad.

As we walk the stone-dust paths, I pick up fallen branches, tossing them over the deer fence toward the wetlands. One client spots an emerging plant.

"Is that poison ivy (*Toxicodendron radicans*)?"

I look and say, "No, you are close; that's Jack-in-the-pulpit (*Arisaema triphyllum*), which looks like poison ivy when small. It's a lovely perennial that has a tall stalk, or spadix, inside a hooded cup. In Fall, a cluster of bright red berries emerge before the plant goes dormant. Next month the spadix should be out."

Most had never heard of this plant but are interested in seeing how it will look next month. We continue our walk until we circle back to the front door of Ann's Place and the start of our class.

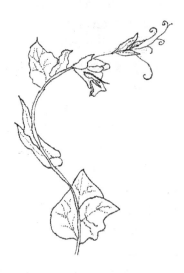

MY MOTHER'S GREENING THUMB

My mother is becoming more active in her garden as the weather has turned. I call her, asking if there are any signs of the lipstick tulips that we had planted last Fall.

"Why yes, Erik. They are flowering and look wonderful."

I should not be surprised. The gardens in Long Island are always a month or so ahead of ours, which are still dormant. I need to drive down from Connecticut to help my mother clean debris from her garden. When I suggest it, she is pleased, looking forward to my visit.

Getting my mother to attend to her garden has been a great solace as she now has an activity that gets her outside to walk and extend her limbs. After my father died, she didn't want to do much save sit in her chair and read one of her many romance novels. Her ability to walk deteriorated and she started to use a cane to steady her gait. But now with a garden, she ventures outside every day to inspect her plantings and often gives me a call on the progress (or lack thereof) of her greenery.

When I arrive at my mother's house a few days later, we visit a local nursery for annuals, finding only pansies (*Viola tricolor* var. *hortensis*) and early-season vegetables to put into the ground. It is too early to get begonias (*Begonia*) and impatiens (*Impatiens walleriana*), which we had planted last year and did wonderfully well. My mother loves pansies, but because of her medical conditions and age she is unable to deadhead the plants after they flower. Between the lack of sun (being on the north side of the house) and the lack of maintenance, her pansies did poorly last year. We decide to ignore the annuals for at least the time being and buy some pine chips and dehydrated manure to dress up and nourish her garden beds, as well as some grass seed to patch some bare spots on the lawn.

When we get home, we take a walk around the garden to look at her tulips. She becomes upset as around a third of them that had recently flowered are missing. "What happened? They were here a few days ago," she says, leaning her cane against the house.

"I'm not sure, Mom, but it seems you have visitors," I reply, pointing at a topped-off tulip stem that was likely consumed by a rabbit. Her facial expressions display disgust, but she accepts the fate of her flowers.

I tell her that those flowers that have not been eaten need deadheading so that they will have a more robust bloom next year. I give her a set of pruners and have her clip off the developing seed heads. It is difficult for her to use this tool, but the task offers a good stretch for her arms and back.

Walking around the yard, my mother wants to seed the bare spots on the lawn. She has arthritis and a difficult time holding items. To help her, I place the grass seed in an unused cookie tin so she can grab small handfuls easily, and I demonstrate how to broadcast it. We work together as a team: I rake the bare spots to disturb the soil, and she then throws down the seed from the tin I am holding.

We make our way around the yard looking for bare spots. She walks over to one place and then backtracks to another. The day becomes warm and sunny and she lingers, sowing the seed slowly as it slips through her thin, arthritic fingers.

After we finish seeding, we take a final walk around the house. The rose bush I had discovered last year in the back of the yard is sending up new shoots around the trellis I erected. The recently planted Japanese maple (*Acer palmatum*) has survived Winter with tiny red leaves emerging from its stems.

My mother notices an old garden bed next to the house where my father used to plant tomatoes (*Solanum lycopersicum*). It is weedy with dandelions (*Taraxacum officinale*), crabgrass (*Digitaria sanguinalis*), and a dead weeping willow tree (*Salix babylonica*) that Juana and I had given them many years ago.

"That really looks horrible," says my mother. "We should do something."

"Well, Mom, we can just pull everything out and leave it for the grass to take over, or we could start another flower garden."

"Let me think about it," she replies as she starts her way back into the house, but not before noticing a random group of daffodils that recently emerged near the back corner of the garage. She bends over carefully to sample their fragrance.

GARDENING IMPROV

My students and I are evicted from the greenhouse at Green Chimneys until certain repairs can be made to it; our carefully planned Spring planting schedule for the Children's Garden needs a quick realignment. This couldn't have come at a more inopportune time as we are just beginning to put the cold-weather vegetables out to harden off and starting to seed the warm weather ones.

"We'll be able to plant just enough to fill the Children's Garden," says Tracy, who runs the horticultural-therapy program here. "But no more than that. Now we need to find new homes for all of our flats. They must be removed from the greenhouse immediately." Luckily we are able to find greenhouse substitutes scattered around the school grounds.

Some seedlings find a home in the tack room of the horse barn, with its large south-facing windows, others over at a neighboring farm, and some in the staff room at the farm. Our composting worms are taking up residency in the livestock barn. They do not require much light. We are forced to begin the hardening process for our vegetables earlier than typical by building additional warm beds, makeshift protective "structures" built from rotting and pungent bales of straw, horse manure, and a cover of spare storm windows that we find in the barn. The work area for my students is moved to an empty (and manure-free) stall in the stables. For the foreseeable future, we will be working outside unless the weather is quite horrible.

It is a raw, windy day with a gray sky and temperatures hovering just around forty degrees. Normally, I would stay inside with my students but we now have work to do that cannot wait.

"Come on, Hugo, we need to reinstall these hoop houses in the garden."

"But Mr. Keller, we took them down last week," he whines.

"I know, but we have had to make a change in plans because we can't use the greenhouse and we need to warm up the soil faster than we thought we needed to last week. I'm sorry, but this is what we must do."

Because it is cold and raw, we work quickly, much faster than in previous outings when the weather was more in tune with the idea and practice of gardening. In about fifteen minutes, we work ourselves into a good sweat as we put the hoops into the ground and then attach the Agribon row covers with clips. A promise of hot chocolate puts Hugo in a better mood to finish his work. Finally, we retreat to the kitchen to warm our hands and stomachs.

By the afternoon, the weather turns as the sun comes out and the day warms. My next group of students weed rows, mulch hostas (*Hosta*), and build a border by the front gates out of rocks we find in the nearby woods. A few carrots (*Daucus carota* var. *sativus*) that were planted last Fall and escaped an earlier harvest are passed around as a treat for a job well done; they are small but sweet to the palate. No one seems to mind that we don't have a greenhouse anymore. We are outside, ready to garden.

APRIL CRAFT: ARRANGE NATURE'S DRIED FLOWERS

April is the month to start tidying up the garden. Though much of the old foliage and leaves belong in the compost pile, many different dried seed pods and flowers can be collected.

The dehydrated flower heads of hydrangeas (Hydrangea) that have been decorating the yard for Winter are a great place to begin. Most varieties are ready to be cut back and the cuttings can be used to form large bouquets. Wild grasses can also be used in a decorative fashion as their seed pods have intriguing patterns and textures. Sea oats (Uniola paniculata) is one of my favorites. And let's not forget perennials like coneflowers (Echinacea) and black-eyed Susan (Rudbeckia hirta), and rose (Rosa) hips. If the birds have not eaten them yet, they all look great in a vase.

PLANTING PEAS AND HANGING STRING

The soil has warmed and it is pea-planting time in the Children's Garden. With my students, I need to plant two rows of peas (*Pisum sativum*), each row about sixty feet long. In a few weeks I will hang strings for the peas to strangle and follow upwards. But first the peas need to get into the soil.

One challenge when working with special-needs children is getting them to plant either seedlings or seeds at a consistent space and depth. While some may believe that this type of rigor is unneeded, part of horticultural therapy is to persuade the child to tap into his or her intelligence, control, and skill. I have found that when you have high expectations in the garden, they will be met often.

This turns out to be the case as I work with Sheila to plant peas. She is slight and shy, hiding her elfin face behind long hair. A chill lingers in the air, so I give her cotton gardening gloves to warm her hands. We then gather our tools.

When a pea is planted, it needs to be inserted between a half and one inch deep into the soil and around two inches from its counterparts so they do not crowd each other. As I have discovered over the years, most children do not have a good concept of inches, and a ruler or tape measure is rarely an effective tool. Instead I fabricate a template and tool for Sheila.

Looking around the grounds I find the perfect tool, a stick, which serves three purposes: It makes a hole, it measures the depth of the hole, and it measures the space needed to plant the peas.

I first cut the stick so that a branch nub is half an inch from the end. By pushing the stick into the ground, Sheila can make a hole for a pea as well as understand how deep to push the stick. I also cut a notch into the stick that is two inches from its other end. I tell Sheila that she needs to space the peas far enough apart so that one pea will touch the end of the stick and the subsequent pea will touch the notch. She nods and we start to plant. I tell her that she is in charge. She will tell me what to do.

Sheila and I start to plant peas with rigor: I hold the peas, she pokes a hole in the soil, I give her the pea, which she drops into a hole, and then I cover the pea up with soil. She soon is bored of this and decides instead to poke ten holes at the same time, fill each with a pea, and then move on. She also wants to hold the peas, leaving me with little to do save place soil on top of each pea once it is in the ground. With each ten feet of row that we plant, she makes subtle but time-saving changes in our chore. By the end of our planting time together, I can barely keep up with her as her work pace accelerates and she is ecstatic with her progress. She is racing to finish. We plant 120 feet of peas in forty minutes.

"I can't believe we did all that work in such a short amount of time. That was fun," says Sheila. Our time together has flown by and soon it is time to return to class. Sheila grabs some greens she finds in the garden and munches them as we walk back, happy with our success and looking forward to working in the garden next week.

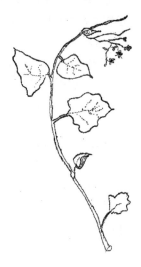

POUNDING LIFE INTO FLOWERS

Smash. Thump. Thwack.

"I can't believe how beautiful this looks!"

"This doesn't look like yours."

"It's better to do it on the floor."

Let me explain. My clients are pounding flowers.

Flower pounding is not an exercise of abuse or violence; it's about expressing the color and pattern of a flower. Most of the clients who arrive at my session at Meadow Ridge, a senior community, do not know what to expect and speculate about the strange request on the sign-up sheet: "Bring a rubber mallet or hammer if you have one."

Shonda comes armed with her mallet, proud that she was able to purchase it for one dollar at a tag sale. "It was a great bargain," she crows while swinging it in hand like an elderly female Thor. As others start to file in, they too are puzzled about what we will be doing but are intrigued, as nearly a dozen pansies, violas (*Viola*), and three large, daisy-like cinerarias (*Pericallis hybrida*) are stationed around the table.

"It's great that so many of you have brought mallets," I say. "It'll make the project so much easier. What we'll be doing today is creating art out of flowers through smashing them with a hammer."

Many peer at me with a skeptical gaze as I pass around samples of flower-pounding art. They are pleasantly surprised at what they see, and as they examine the pictures, I describe how to pound flowers.

"Everyone gets two pieces of paper to create their impressions. First you place the flower face down on your watercolor paper, keeping in mind you want to spread the petals. Next you cover it with a paper towel and then pound away a few times." To demonstrate, I grab a pansy flower, place it face down on the watercolor paper, cut off the back stem so that it will flatten better, cover it, and smack it with a hammer.

When I pull away the paper towel, I discover that the image transferred to the watercolor paper is muddy and incomplete. Nuts. Not at all like other pansy prints I have created. What did I do wrong?

As I sheepishly reveal my image to the class, I surmise that the problem may be with the table. It is a wobbly plastic affair that flexes and moves as I wallop the flower. I make another attempt with a different flower on the corner of the table, which has better support.

When I remove the paper towel after this pounding, a perfect image shows up on the watercolor paper. Oohs and ahs follow. Success! It is now my clients' turn.

Some clients are tentative in smacking the flowers hard, as arthritic and weak hands make the task more difficult. But they find that many tiny taps instead will transfer the flower pattern to paper if they are patient. Others swing their hammers with abandon, preferring to make a single smack to affect the transfer from flower to paper. Talking is difficult as the pounding fills the room with sound.

"Can we pound the leaves?" asks Sharon over the din.

"The viola leaves don't transfer well but I don't know about the cinerarias," I reply.

That motivates Sharon to remove a leaf and give it a good smack. The result is vivid, not only showing the green of the leaf but also its venation.

Even the efforts that are incomplete have a beauty to them. And we have the opportunity to augment Nature with Sharpies and colored pencils.

Molly's first attempts produce an image that is not pleasing to her. "This doesn't look right," she says. "Don't worry about the first image," I counsel. "It's the composite of all your attempts that will define your art. Try pounding another flower on top to create an image of a bouquet."

Stephanie is becoming, in the words of a friend, "the teacher's pet." She composes a beautiful mosaic of flowers, making some appear to pop out of the page. Soon everyone has a portrait they are proud of. Though we have only a few types of flowers and just a couple of colors, everyone creates unique images that they are happy with. When I tell everyone to take a pansy plant back to their apartment, it is a bonus that few expect.

APRIL OUTING: TURN OVER OLD LEAVES

Leaf litter is still heavy on the ground as the warmth needed to turn it into humus has yet to arrive. But wonderful discoveries can be made underneath Nature's blanket with simple and gentle turns. Fern fronds are starting to emerge as are a myriad of weeds, some of which can be tasty to sample, such as garlic mustard and wild spinach (Chenopodium album).

Plants aren't the only things waking up. A careful turning of the leaves or logs can reveal a dormant tree frog or salamander whose natural antifreeze keeps them alive during Winter. They should not be disturbed but marveled at from afar.

HARVEST AND SNIFF

Herbs are not usually ready for harvest in April, but this morning as Selma and I clean a few of the raised beds in the Children's Garden, we find ourselves in the middle of a smell-a-thon. It is early in the morning with the sun beginning to rise and melt the light frost, which hangs off the plants and Agribon hoop houses. It is brisk but windless. Selma and I need to ready a bed for planting that holds a patch of wintered-over cilantro (*Coriandrum sativum*). Last November we built a hoop house around the patch because it had self-seeded and looked too good to just let die. Even after a snow-laden Winter with little attention, it greened up last month and small amounts were ready for use a few weeks ago.

We remove the Agribon fabric and a waft of heat and cilantro-scented air greets us. Though chilly outside, the soil is warm and moist within the confines of the hoop house.

"How is this possible?" asks Selma. "It was just Winter a few weeks ago."

One of the things that pleases me about our gardens is how we have been able to fool Nature (and some of our children) by extending the seasons and times we have been able to work in the garden. From harvesting lettuce (*Lactuca sativa*) in December to carrots in January to turnip greens (*Brassica rapa* subsp. *rapa*) in March, we have been able to show how the garden is alive with plants year round.

We prune the bottom of the cilantro and place it into a bucket. Selma huddles toward one side of the row as the heat rising from the soil helps keep her warm. At first she wants to wear gloves, but I suggest to her that it will be more fun to use her bare hands to better appreciate the scent of the herbs. She doesn't understand until I tell her to smell her fingers after a few cuttings. She does and a big smile frames her face. Selma comes to life as the scent of cilantro envelops her. Our progress slows as she can't help smelling her hands to take in the fragrance. We harvest a pound of the herb; it will be sent to the school kitchen to be used for meals.

We then move to an area in the garden dedicated to perennial herbs, including thyme (*Thymus vulgaris*), sage (*Salvia officinalis*), oregano (*Origanum vulgare*), mint, and lavender (*Lavandula angustifolia*). The sun has yet to fully warm this area, and a blanket of frost still covers many of the herbs, encased in a dull white sheen. We need to trim the thyme, which has escaped its bed and is beginning to enter the walking path.

I tell Selma to cut a line with her pruners straight across the bed's edge, so that the thyme appears as a fuzzy border on top of the bed's wooden rail. The thyme is now thick and woody, making any cutting very difficult. After a few attempts, she drops the pruners and looks as if she is going to cry.

"Selma, don't worry. Take a break and smell the herbs," I counsel. "You'll feel better." I give her some of the thyme she was trying to cut as well as lavender and mint.

"What do they remind you of?" I ask, watching her calm herself while smelling the herbs. She cannot recall exactly.

"This reminds me of home," she says, after a pause, holding up the lavender.

"Perhaps your mother or grandmother used to have a perfume that they would wear," I suggest. "Or maybe a soap that you used or they had at home." She perks up. "Yes, that's it. Could I smell a bit more?"

While Selma lingers over the plants, I trim the thyme. Soon she is ready to get back to work. When her hands tire, she goes back to the lavender for a sniff and remembrance of things past. She appears peaceful and reflective, unworried about her inability to cut certain sprigs of the thyme. We divide the task: I cut the heavier, thick stems, Selma the light, thin ones. After we finish, we take our buckets of thyme and cilantro to the kitchen. I give her a little sprig of lavender and Selma keeps it near her nose for most of the walk back to her class.

WHEN STUDENTS PULL AWAY

One of my favorite students that I have worked with in the Children's Garden is Seymour. Seymour is an exceptionally bright child with a variety of emotional challenges. We had hit it off last year, as he loves carnivorous plants; I have a pretty good knowledge of them because I propagate them. This mutual interest formed an initial bond and intense working relationship unlike ones that I had with other children. Seymour was driven. It seemed that nothing was too challenging for him as we worked through the garden on a variety of chores.

This hard work and good behavior culminated in Seymour's receiving a Cape sundew (*Drosera capensis*) plant at the end of November after working with me for three months successfully. I remember his pride and happiness when I gave him the plant and built a shelf for him in his room so he could place it near a window. Seymour was doing really well and appeared responsible enough to take care of an exotic plant. It pleased me to be able to give Seymour a plant he could care for.

Then something happened.

After the New Year, I was not allowed to work with Seymour anymore. "Seymour is having some problems," I was told when I went by to pick him up from class. "He can't garden today."

This continued for the entire Winter academic session, so I didn't see him for more than three months. When I went to his teacher recently to see if I could reengage with him, I was told no and that he had just been transferred to a class for students with more acute challenges. No more jobs for Seymour. No more gardening.

Last week, Seymour saw me across the campus and ran over. "Mr. Keller, when are you coming to pick me up for my garden job?" he asked.

"You don't have a garden job anymore, Seymour."

"Why not?"

"You tell me. A gardening job is a privilege. Have you been behaving in school and staying out of trouble so you can be rewarded with a job?" Silence. "And what happened to the Cape sundew I gave you? That was your baby."

"They took it away from me," he said, looking deflated and a bit ashamed.

"Well, there must have been a good reason, Seymour. But I'll make a deal with you, if you can turn things around, do your schoolwork, take care of your room, and get along with your fellow students, I will talk to your teachers to see if you can get back your old job."

For now, Seymour is not getting any better.

While this is an extreme example, there are other smaller ones reminding me of the children's fragility. A few weeks ago, George and I were planting peas. Everything seemed fine; he worked well in the garden and was happy to be doing such a great job. A few hours later I found him curled up leaning against a wall crying inconsolably while two adults were trying to comfort him. Another student I recently started with missed his last two sessions; I learned that he needed to be taken to a different acute-care facility.

One of the wonderful aspects of horticultural therapy is that it takes its participants to very different places. The garden is a healing place that gives children a different and positive place to learn and grow. Every so often, however, I am reminded that life is no garden for all children.

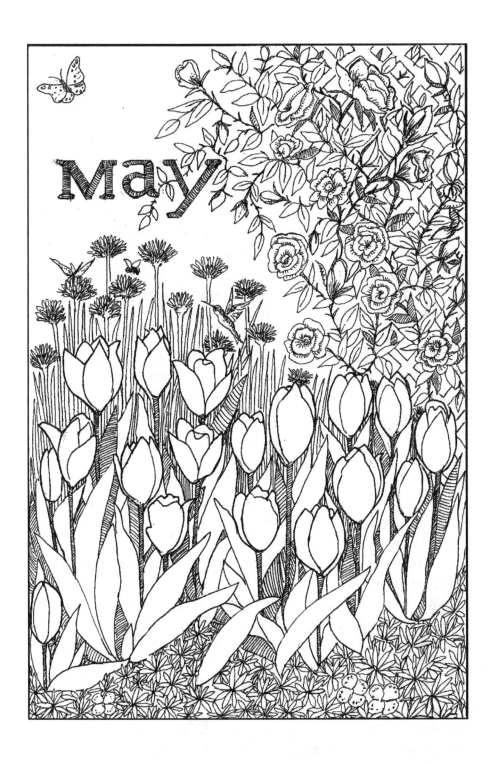

MAY: FLOWER TIME

May is the transition month in New England for gardens. Pent up growth bursts forth, and it is no coincidence that indigenous Americans called the full moon of this month the Flower Moon. Spring greens, radishes (Raphanus sativus), and peas (Pisum sativum) become abundant at farm stands, and tulips (Tulipa) and young roses (Rosa) bloom with color.

It is also the time when the first weeds of the season make a big push to flower and seed quickly to perpetuate themselves. Many of the migrating birds have returned from the South, and skunks have emerged from their Winter lairs ready to breed. The garden is exploding with life.

FOOD FOR HARVEST AND REFLECTION

The first major harvest is upon us in the Children's Garden. The mustard greens (*Brassica juncea*) wintered over nicely in their hoop house. When we peeled off the Agribon fabric last month, they had just come out of their dormancy, their shriveled leaves abandoned for fresh shoots. Now, a month later, the large-leafed, dark green plants are going to seed and must be harvested.

Jeff and I remove the leaves from the stems so Tracy can deliver them to the food pantry later today. Jeff is attentive but melancholy. His grandfather died recently. He and his father have been cleaning out his grandfather's house over the last month, and he wants to tell me about all the things they have found. "My grandpa had a 2002 Chevy that we're going to take home," he says. "We're going to store it in the backyard, and I'll be getting it when I turn eighteen." Jeff is eleven years old. He abruptly tells me that he doesn't want to speak anymore of his grandfather, so we work together quietly and I give him lots of space.

Jeff carefully picks each mustard leaf off each stem and asks how the leaves are used to make mustard, which he enjoys on hot dogs. I tell him that the leaves are used for salads while the seeds are ground into mustard. "See the little yellow flower? That will form a seed, which can then be made into mustard."

"Can I eat one?" he asks. "No problem," I reply. He bites into the leaf and almost immediately his mouth puckers up and eyes squint. Jeff spits out the leaf. Too bitter. I ask if his grandfather liked mustard. Jeff looks up and slowly replies, "Yes, on hot dogs. He would make them for me when we barbecued during Summer." He sighs quietly and a small tear wells up in his left eye. We stop talking and he goes back to the harvest. We collect a large pile of mustard greens that weighs two pounds and put it in the refrigerator so it can be delivered later to the local food pantry.

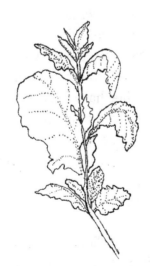

TURNING A BLACK THUMB INTO A GREEN ONE

My mother was never an active gardener, though she loves flowers. In Spring I bring her cut lilac flowers (*Syringa vulgaris*) from my garden and she revels in their fragrance. It is one of her favorite scents, and it fills the kitchen after she places the flowers in her favorite vase. But she feels quite different when I bring her a living plant. She looks at me in a pleasing manner, but with a sigh of resignation says, "Well, you know Erik, this is just going to die. I have a black thumb."

Now, my mother is not the type of person who actively cuts the blooms off roses, as Morticia Addams would, but she has had a knack for transforming luscious green plants into crumbling brown ones. This is hard to believe from a woman who as a young girl spent Summers at her uncle Bill and aunt Ruth Johnston's farm, getting up before dawn to feed and water the chickens and tend to the vegetable gardens.

One year in late Spring, we needed to go to a local nursery store on Long Island to pick up some peat moss. My mother initially didn't want to leave the car, but I convinced her it would be good just to get out to stretch her legs. She agreed and soon was meandering around all the different flowers that were on display. She appeared to enter another world, as she was smiling and gently touching different plants. The pansies (*Viola tricolor* var. *hortensis*) were soon in her sights. "I love pansies," she said, "but they always die on me." She felt the petals gently and sniffed a nearby purple lilac.

This Spring I decide to reintroduce my mother to her gardens. The easiest place to start is the two flower beds that flank the front door. As long as I can remember, they have been a horticultural wasteland, a death sentence for anything that was planted, save a pair of mangy boxwoods (*Buxus*) bracketing this inhospitable area between the garage and the western edge of the house. After examining the space in some detail, I finally understand why. There is no soil in the ground to nourish plants, only leftover construction dirt, sand, and concrete pieces.

Making matters more challenging for any plant, the beds are located on the north side of the house and get little sunlight and even less rain water, because an overhang from the roof keeps most of the area bone dry. Even weeds keep their distance. We have some work in front of us if we want to get plants to grow. My mother is not enthusiastic initially but is willing to attempt a change, so we go to a local gardening center.

We first buy large bags of soil, compost, and dehydrated manure. "Do we really need all this stuff?" asks my mother. I assure her that we need it all. We then buy some plants. My mother insists that we buy pansies, even though I know it is unlikely that they would thrive on the shaded north side of the house. As we walk toward the register to pay for our goods, my mother lingers around the tuberous begonias (*Begonia tuberhybrida*). "These are lovely," she says. We purchase a dark red one, load up the car, and head home.

Along with our purchases, we have some plants I dug up from my yard, including hostas (*Hosta*), astilbes (*Astilbe*), bleeding hearts (*Lamprocapnos spectabilis*), and ferns (*Tracheophyta*). These are all hardy and will do well in the shade. I bring them near the front stoop where my mother can look at them. She has a hard time crouching or kneeling, so she sits on the front steps directing me where to dig. She quickly sees the poor condition of the beds, and she notes the difference between the sand and construction debris and the bags of new organic material.

"Mom, smell the difference. Feel it." She looks at me quizzically but tentatively takes a handful each of her dirt and the purchased soil. The brown-black soil is thick, moist, and can be compressed with a hand squeeze. Her dirt, on the other hand, is a nondescript color, dry and lifeless. She is beginning to understand the difference.

We work together, me digging out the dirt and her handing me pots of soil, compost, and manure to mix in a hole. I put in the plants. My mother removes the pansies from their cell packs and spreads the roots. This is a good exercise for her arthritic fingers. She enjoys splitting up the plants, though later she remarks about how long it takes to get the soil out from under her fingernails.

In a little more than an hour, we plant the two garden beds adjacent to the front door. After I spread dark brown mulch around all the plants, my mother waters everything down with a good soaking. It would have been easier to put on a sprinkler, but I wanted her to experience standing over them with a garden hose to care for them. We enjoy the dinner that she prepares for me, and as dusk approaches I drive home to Connecticut.

As I check in on her in the weeks to come, an amazing thing happens. She waters all the time. She pinches her spent pansy blooms. The front garden now has flowers.

I call my mother a couple of times a week, and we often talk about the garden and how it is doing. Everyday, even during days it rains, my mother checks the garden to see if the soil is dry.

Everything is growing well (except for one astilbe that didn't take). Later in the season we add dark red impatiens (*Impatiens walleriana*). My mother loves dark red flowers. Many of her neighbors and friends have told her how beautiful her garden looks now. She is very proud; she is even thinking about letting me start another bed in the back of the house, which gets sun all day.

CHANGES IN ATTITUDE AND SPIDER HOMES

I am looking forward to picking up Cheryl, as there is much to do in the Children's Garden; the lettuce (*Lactuca sativa*) has started to bolt, or go to seed, and the spinach (*Spinacia oleracea*) is ready for harvest. When I pick her up I notice that something's not right. Cheryl is looking at one of the classroom computers intently, and when I say it is time for her to work in the garden she protests, "I don't want to go! I hate being in the garden." She is not given a choice, so she grabs her coat and with a huff and sulky disposition follows me out.

Strolling toward the garden, I ask her how her week has gone and how she feels. "It has been horrible and things suck," she replies, choking back a few tears. We stop and rest on a nearby bench. Her feet dangle and she looks down toward the ground.

"Is there anything you want to do in the garden?" I ask.

"No," she says.

"Would you like to talk?"

"No."

A similar problem occurred with Cheryl a month ago, and I took her back to class rather than risk her having a breakdown in the garden. Unfortunately, that decision may not have been the best, as her subsequent returns to the garden have turned into power struggles that make her more upset and agitated. I try a different approach this time.

"Cheryl, we will be harvesting spinach and lettuce. Would you like to see the peas we planted last month before we begin?"

"No."

We walk to the barn to get kneeling pads and pruning shears. With few words exchanged, we sit down in front of the lettuce and I show her how to harvest it using pruners. Cheryl takes the pruners from me and works intermittently with a far-away look on her face as she cuts the leaves and places them in a bin. I work next to her, weeding an adjacent patch. She remains emotionless as she rhythmically cuts the plants; after a while, she begins to relax. Her face softens. Suddenly she notices a butterfly.

"What type of butterfly is that?" she asks.

"It looks like a swallowtail, but I am not sure," I reply. "It is looking for a flower so it can have a snack."

"Does it eat the flower?" Cheryl inquires. "No," I say. "Butterflies sip the nectar of plants with their straw-like tongues. If we have flowers in the garden, butterflies and other bugs will come to eat and pollinate. Let's try to take a closer look."

We put our pruners down and walk slowly over to the flower that the butterfly—it is a swallowtail—is resting upon. It is indifferent to our presence, and Cheryl and I watch it take long drinks with its proboscis. After it flies away, we return to our chores. Cheryl is now more animated and content. By the time we have finished cutting lettuce, she is smiling and happy with her work. "I'm done," she says with pride in her voice.

"No you aren't," I tease. "You missed one."

In the middle of the cut lettuce patch is a tiny, uncut floret. I snip it with my shears and give it to her. "Try it."

Her eyes open up as she bites into it. "That's awesome! It's so delicious!" she exclaims.

I smile and ask her to pick up our harvest so we can weigh it. I marvel at the change in Cheryl; she went from depression to extreme happiness.

Weighing the harvest, I grab some leaves and hold them to her nose. The fresh smell is powerful and slightly sweet. Cheryl loves it. "I never smelled anything like that," she says.

"So what does it smell like?" I ask.

She thinks about it for a while and replies that she doesn't know.

"It smells like lettuce, you silly goose," I say. She laughs and smiles.

We move on to the spinach where she has excellent focus. She eats a leaf and is surprised by its taste. But mostly she is shocked by its size. "These are humongous," she says. We then have a contest to see who can find the largest spinach leaf. She wins, but not before she accidentally rips the winning leaf. Cheryl wants to fix it using scotch tape, but I tell her that most people would not like tape as part of their dinner. "They could always take it off. It would look pretty," she laughs.

Finishing our chores, I notice a lone head of lettuce in an adjacent row. It hadn't been cut because we found a large brown spider that had taken up residence inside. "Do you think the spider is still there?" asks Cheryl, remembering why we had left it. I pull away some leaves but find no sign of the arachnid, so we clip and add it to our pile. For the morning, we have harvested nearly ten pounds of food.

It turns out I am not a good spider inspector. Soon our brown spider climbs out of the cut lettuce carrying a large fluffy white ball. "What's that?" asks Cheryl.

"That is the spider's egg nest. She is getting ready to have babies."

Because the spider is a mother, Cheryl is not fast to ask me to kill it, as is often the case when we come across spiders. So I place the spider and her egg nest on a fence post.

"Cheryl, have you ever read the story *The Very Busy Spider*?"

"Yes, it's one of my favorites."

"Mine too," I reply as we spend the remainder of our time talking about spiders, rats, barns, and humongous spinach leaves.

BABY FOOD

Charlotte and I go often to my garden for a morning snack. We have a routine. She walks up the steps of the old greenhouse foundation where my raised beds sit, pausing to pat the black ceramic frog next to the gate. She then takes her finger and traces out the initials of her name spelled in the stones that I mortared onto the foundation a little after she was born.

Earlier in the season she turned to the right to make a grab at some lettuce, which was plentiful in the cold frame. Now she turns left looking for strawberries (*Fragaria ×ananassa*), walking along a narrow walkway between the raised strawberry bed and a small greenhouse. The strawberries are tiny, green, and have not yet matured. Every day she hopes to spot a fat red one but continues to be disappointed. No matter, she knows that they will be ready for her to sample soon.

If she doesn't turn into the greenhouse to rearrange the pots, she then heads over a narrow walkway next to the sorrel (*Rumex acetosa*). Grabbing a leaf or two and stuffing them into her mouth has become second nature for her as she surveys the rest of the garden. To the right are a few tomato (*Solanum lycopersicum*) plants that I put into the garden early and from which delicate flowers are emerging. Charlotte has yet to discover that these will become one of her favorite plants in Summer, once their delectable tiny pear tomatoes begin to ripen. Next to the tomatoes are different types of lettuce that she grabs occasionally. I need to be more diligent when inspecting the leaves— they have become second homes to the emerging slug population.

While munching away, Charlotte picks up a soap-shaped rock in the bird bath and puts it down several times while splashing her other hand in the water. When she attempts to lick the rock, I divert her attention to other parts of the garden.

We tickle each other's noses with sprigs of thyme (*Thymus vulgaris*) and oregano (*Origanum vulgare*) that are in abundance. She gives up an expansive grin and chuckles to her Pampi (me). We then make our last stop at the snow peas (*Pisum sativum* var. *saccharatum*) that are climbing up a trellis. I give Charlotte a pod or two and she looks them over before sticking one into her mouth. A satisfying crunch follows.

She knows it is time to leave the garden and explore other areas of the yard. I help her up over the step from the rear of the garden, and she walks to the gate, signaling for my hand.

MAY CRAFT: HERBAL HANGING BASKETS

May is just the best time of year to create hanging baskets. Inexpensive cell packs of herbs are available and ready for planting. If you wait until the end of the month, choices can be limited, and if it gets too hot during the month, all the packs in the stores will have bolted. Larger hanging baskets can accommodate three different types of herbs, but in those cases you need to trim them diligently so they don't overgrow the basket. In addition, the taller herbs like basil (Ocimum basilicum) should be placed in the middle of the basket so they do not shade low-growing herbs like thyme.

Herb plants from nurseries can often be divided into multiple seedlings to make more than one basket from a single purchase. You can start them from seeds now, but then you would be waiting until mid to late Summer before you have a chance to use them in your recipes.

CLIENT BALANCE

A few years ago one of my younger students in the Children's Garden came up with a great idea. She had read about the poverty and hunger that afflicts children around the world. She said that it would be wonderful if we could grow vegetables in the Children's Garden for those less fortunate. Her selfless idea has become a yearly project. One year we harvested more than one hundred pounds of food that was donated to a local food pantry from a single row of three by thirty-five feet. And now it is time for another donation.

The morning is clear and crisp as we remove the Agribon cover from the row to reveal lushly growing romaine lettuce (*Lactuca sativa* var. *longifolia*), arugula (*Eruca vesicaria* subsp. *sativa*), parsley (*Petroselinum crispum*), and spinach. The warm weather along with frequent rains have accelerated their growth, giving us the opportunity for an early harvest.

The radishes, broccoli (*Brassica oleracea* var. *italica*), and carrots (*Daucus carota* subsp. *sativus*), however, have not yet matured, a problem we seem to be having in other garden rows with similar vegetables. As we fold the Agribon away from its hoops, Malik wants to know why we cover the plants.

"It keeps them warm," I reply.

"Then why are we taking the cloth off?" my young charge retorts.

"Well, do you stay in bed all day?" I ask.

"No, it would be too hot under the blankets," he answers.

I smile. "Plants are the same."

Today we will harvest half the arugula and lettuce. Surveying our row, I can't help but feel proud that my students are helping to feed less fortunate people in a neighboring town.

To create this garden, my students and I worked closely together to ensure we have straight rows of aligned plants. Unlike many of the other rows in the Children's Garden, which are not organized rigidly, for these I have taken clues from Mel Bartholomew's classic book *Square Foot Gardening* to teach my students to plant tightly and with exactness. I often give students here much leeway to encourage independent thought and action. But when we are working to feed the poor, some of this goes by the wayside, and I maintain tighter control over the planting to maximize yield.

For some children, this approach is especially helpful, as their actions and thoughts are spontaneous, and without such control they would be inattentive. By paying close attention to each child, I hope to serve both clients—the ones who need the food as well as the ones who need guidance and understanding.

Malik and I wash out a blue plastic tub with white rope handles for the greens. I tell Malik to cut the romaine lettuce so we harvest a head rather than single leaves. He has difficulty with the first half dozen or so heads, sometimes cutting too high, other times too low and in the soil. With some careful guidance, however, Malik is soon able to cut the lettuce like a pro, removing nicely cut heads from the garden with a minimum of soil. When weighed, we have five pounds of romaine.

The arugula is different, as we need to just cut the leaves. This comes more naturally to Malik and he quickly and enthusiastically gathers what we need for the day. We add one pound of arugula to the day's harvest.

Malik is pleased that the lettuce grows so quickly. He and I planted seedlings only a month ago. After we finish our chores, we walk over to the asparagus (*Asparagus officinalis*) patch, and I cut a new shoot for him to eat. He knows that we don't have that much asparagus and a spear is a real treat this time of year.

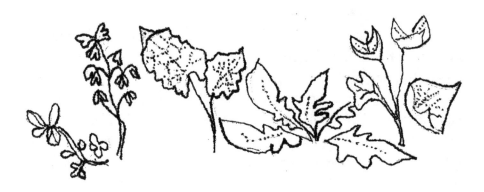

EATING ON THE WILD SIDE

The rains and warming temperatures of the season bring new growth to both wanted and unwanted plants. The growth of unwanted plants or weeds always seems to outpace that of the more desirable cultivars. But a weed is just a plant that you don't want in a particular place. With this in mind, I hope to change the perspective of a few adults at Ann's Place about the edible greens that are common in yards and gardens this time of year.

While the advantages of eating local produce and food are becoming increasingly popular, the most local way to eat is from what is growing in your backyard. Time to forage. This is an easy class to prep for as my yard is replete with traditional weeds: burdock (*Arctium*), chive (*Allium schoenoprasum*), clover (*Trifolium*), dandelion (*Taraxacum officinale*), garlic mustard (*Alliaria petiolata*), mint (*Mentha*), broadleaf plantain (*Plantago major*), Queen Anne's lace (*Daucus carota*), sheep sorrel (*Rumex acetosella*), sweet woodruff (*Galium odoratum*), violets (*Viola*), wild garlic (*Allium ursinum*), wild onion (*Allium canadense*), and wild creeping thyme (*Thymus serpyllum*). I gather them up and prepare them for my clients to ingest later.

The class starts with a walk into the backyard of Ann's Place. The diverse edible plants I find here are a mix of sweet and tangy greens as well as different herbs that will freshen up any dish with unfamiliar flavors. About half of them are the same plants that I collected earlier at my house. After showing my clients how to identify, spot, and harvest potential salad additions, they come back ready to sample the greens I have collected.

I offer them a taste of each different leaf and the group is divided, with half deciding to take a chance while the other half demurring politely. Perhaps I should not have told them first that poison hemlock (*Conium maculatum*), which was used to kill Socrates, has a similar appearance to Queen Anne's lace. It is easy, though, to tell them apart—Queen Anne's lace has hairy stems and a root that smells like a carrot; hemlock has smooth stems and the disturbed leaves smell musty or like mouse urine. I caution them about foraging in the wild, as there are a variety of very poisonous plants out in the yard, well described in Amy Stewart's excellent book *Wicked Plants*.

I lay out the different "weeds" on a table for identification. "This first one, burdock, is a delicacy in Asia. The tap root is cooked. But the small leaves can be used in a salad while the larger ones are sautéed," I say. "Historically this has been used as a diuretic as well as a remedy for skin problems.

"If you are not very, very sure of what you are ingesting, don't take a chance. Also, don't harvest food from areas that have just been sprayed with a pesticide or herbicide."

In response to that warning, all are intrigued with the scents of the different plants on display; no harm in smelling. I had clipped a mint from our property that my mother-in-law had smuggled in from Guatemala many years ago. It has a very strong minty scent and a bright purple stalk. "It is really best used for chicken soup," says my wife, Juana, who attends the session along with my granddaughter, Charlotte. Each client takes a sample cutting of the Guatemalan mint to start their own plant at home.

"Cultivated sorrel is a great addition to salads if you want a bit of a kick," I say. "Another name for it is lemon leaf, because of the flavor. And it is a favorite with kids." Almost on cue, Charlotte reaches over to stuff one in her mouth. I then get out the salad I prepared at home from backyard weeds. It contains a wide variety of tiny leaves in different shades of green and textures; I have topped them with magenta redbud (*Cercis canadensis*) flowers. Nearly every client takes a small sample salad that is dressed with a very light vinaigrette. As a group they are surprised and pleased.

"This is wonderful!"

"The flowers taste like snow peas with a sharp aftertaste."

"Can I have some more?"

After we finish off the salad, I offer May wine, a traditional German drink to celebrate May Day as well as the coming of Spring. As I open the carafe I let each client smell the mix of sweet woodruff, strawberries, and Riesling wine. "This is amazing," says Nora. All are smiling in anticipation.

"Now be careful when you drink this, as it does have a reputation as an aphrodisiac," I say. They all smile at me and take their first sip. No one is displeased.

MAY OUTING: VISIT GARDEN CENTERS

May is the best time of year to frequent garden centers. In the Northeast most of the tender annuals have arrived and plants are ready to go into the ground. Many nurseries, particularly those in big box stores, rush the process. Tomatoes, peppers (Capsicum annuum), and other plants that cannot take a frost have been available for over a month. I find no advantage to placing such plants in the ground early; better to keep them inside, in a greenhouse or cold frame until Memorial Day.

Everything else is ready for planting, particularly perennials, bushes, and trees. Now is the time to get them into the ground before the hot and potentially dry heat of Summer hits. Walking around the garden center with an open mind and agenda lets you consider the possibilities. Take some pictures of your house and garden with you so that you can imagine how different plants will fit in. And let your mind go wild.

NEW BATCH OF SEEDLINGS

New seedlings at Ann's Place have made their way into my care. One is a student who is pursuing her certificate in horticultural therapy from the NYBG and the other is a group of special-needs young adults. They both share many characteristics in that they have a lot to learn, want to spend as much time with plants as possible, and hope to develop good work habits and skills to become productive in their chosen fields. But as do a cactus (*Echinopsis*) and Venus fly trap (*Dionaea muscipula*), they have very different care requirements.

Donna, my intern, wants to learn about the craft of horticultural therapy and has just started participating in my classes. Unlike my clients, Donna takes notes frenetically between exercises and activities, recording my steps (and missteps). We chat before and after our sessions so that I can get tips from her on how I can improve, and she can ask me questions about what I did and why during class.

My other charges have different challenges, as they are attempting to become attentive, good workers. This is much harder for special-needs adults as I am taxed to make things interesting for them as well as give them work lessons that they will retain. Unlike Donna, whose tutelage is constant and regular, my special-needs students have vastly different dispositions that can change within minutes.

"Let's remove all of these types of plants from this area," I say to Judy, giving her a plant of mugwort (*Artemisia vulgaris*) as an example. She nods but I'm not sure if she is interested. She starts by following instructions but within minutes becomes distracted and tired of weeding. She starts removing plants that are not weeds.

"What's the problem?" I ask.

"This is boring and I'm tired," Judy replies.

"Well, I know, but we need to weed and this is a job that needs to be done. How about you weed over in the shade, and I will do it in the sun. And then when we are finished, I'll let you mow the lawn with the lawn mower."

"That would be okay," she says.

These students do not absorb my lessons readily but rather require multiple catalysts and redirections to become engaged in an activity. They are trying to learn skills and patience so that they can get a paying job and become somewhat independent. I also find that, as I perceive impending inattention, if I interrupt the activities with different lessons or observations it helps them remain focused on their respective tasks. I show them fiddlehead ferns (*Matteuccia struthiopteris*), edible weeds, toads, groundhog holes, and other discoveries to break the repetition of their jobs.

I remove a spent daffodil (*Narcissus*) pod from a stem and slice it open, revealing a seed factory holding collections of little seeds in concentric rows. "You want to cut these pods off so that all the energy of the plant goes into feeding the bulb, making it bigger so that it will give larger flowers next year and possibly divide to produce more plants. But don't remove the leaves. The bulb needs them to produce energy using photosynthesis for next year's flower."

The students look at the dissected pod with wonder. "That's so cool, why does that happen?" I then discuss how flowers are fertilized, how plants use the energy of the sun for photosynthesis, and soon we are back removing weeds.

It's that sense of wonder and surprise that is really important to impart to a client. I tell Donna, "One of the things I always try to do is surprise and even shock clients. Remember that everyone wants to have fun. Think of it as a joke: you always want to deliver a good punch line."

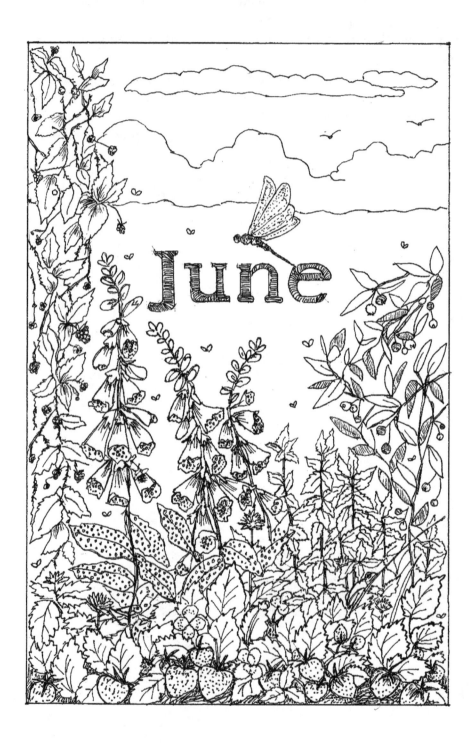

JUNE: SUMMER AWAITS

Snow and frosts have long since faded, flowers are in full bloom, and the vegetable garden has seen harvests. Warm days are frequent and alfresco dinners have begun. Daylight stretches late into the evening with bats emerging at dusk to feast on insects.

The only disadvantage accompanying the explosion of plants is that of bugs. The early gnats of Spring are replaced by a larger and more substantial set of biting insects. But it seems a small price to pay as fresh strawberries (Fragaria ×ananassa*) and highbush blueberries (*Vaccinium corymbosum*) come into their own.*

GROWING TEMPTATION

It can seem like an insurmountable task to get young children to appreciate the nuances of different types of mints (*Mentha*) or to sample a simple chive (*Allium schoenoprasum*). But that effort to impart a new sensation or experience must be part of any gardening or horticultural-therapy program to help illustrate that all the weeding, composting, watering, weeding, planting, weeding, thinning, and tilling is worth it. The end result must be connected with all of the earlier steps.

That is why we built the Children's Garden at Green Chimneys to be diverse and different to astound the senses. It's not just about having a hollyhock (*Alcea*), or marigold (*Tagetes*), or tomato (*Solanum lycopersicum*) in the soil. It's about growing weird and uncommon plants like cosmic purple carrots (*Daucus carota* 'Cosmic

Purple'), Chinese red noodle beans (*Vigna unguiculata* subsp. *sesquipedalis*), or speckled roman tomatoes that will excite and astound multiple senses in students. Visually interesting plants and fruits are just the first step. If you are working with vegetables and flowers, you want to get your charges to love what they do and eat what they grow in the garden. You want them to channel their inner rabbit.

That is why after garden chores, we take the children shopping throughout the garden. We have just finished harvesting all the asparagus (*Asparagus officinalis*) and have started to thin the carrots (*Daucus carota*). For children who are unaccustomed to or unfamiliar with fresh-out-of-the-garden vegetables, it is a wonderful new experience. Most will try anything, though first attempts can be tentative. Their faces soon brighten up, however, when they chomp down on an asparagus shoot that was cut only moments before.

The string-like root structures of fledgling carrots have a barely discernible sweetness. Still, students enjoy nibbling away at what they can gather in the garden. Chives and their flowers have a very different albeit strong flavor. Such strong tastes are attractive. Sorrel (*Rumex acetosa*) and gooseberries (*Ribes uva-crispa*), both of which are very pungent, are favorites. The astringent and sour flavors of both are an acquired taste. Most children will pop a dozen gooseberries into their mouths if you give them the chance.

Garlic (*Allium sativum*) scapes, the tender stem and flower bud of a hard neck garlic bulb, have started to emerge between the leaves, and it is amusing to see the change in expression as a child first bites into one. You do a silent count in your head and when you get to "three Mississippi," their faces explode with the realization that they have bitten into an intense, tangy, hot thing. Some keep chomping, others look to drink a trough of water. But for many of our crops, we need to ration such samplings or our rows would be stripped quickly by a swarm of T-shirt-wearing locusts.

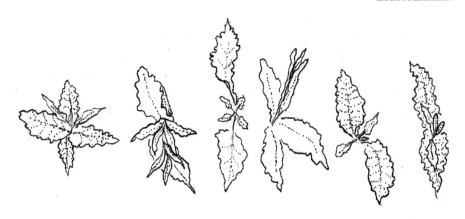

MINTY FRESH WITH A TWIST

A sneaky way to surprise clients is by tapping into seemingly insignificant differences to amplify the breadth and depth of what Nature has to offer. I did that recently with mints and geraniums (*Pelargonium*). I gathered thirteen different ones and a lone Cleveland sage (*Salvia clevelandii*) and set them out on a table with only a letter for identification.

Entering the art room at Ann's Place, my clients are hit with a huge diversity of scents and a few are taken aback by the bouquet. "That is quite heady," says Johanna. "Yeah," I reply. "Think about how my car smells when I come over here."

The sense of smell is often taken for granted but can be very powerful. It can trigger strong emotions. One client talks about her mother's rose (*Rosa*) garden. Her voice cracks a bit and her eyes water as she tells the class of her mom. A neighbor offers a reassuring hug.

"My mother loves lilac flowers (*Syringa vulgaris*)," I add. "I bring them to her every Spring at the nursing home where she now lives. She buries her face into them thinking back to when she was a young girl." My clients nod in understanding. After a few more remembrances by others, I start the class.

"We have fourteen different plants here, each with a different smell. They are gooseberry, lemon-rose, lime, rose, and snowflake geraniums; apple, "chicken-soup," curly, grapefruit, mojito, mountain, mystery, and Ridgefield (peppermint) mints; and a Cleveland sage.

The point of the exercise is not to identify all the different mints precisely but explore the differences.

"Do your best to understand what type of plant it is first and then focus on the characteristics of its smell when compared to others. Also, you might want to wash your hands after smelling a plant or two, as the essential oils of one plant will linger and confuse the smell of the next one."

With that clients start to rub leaves. They love the smelly surprises each plant throws off but after sampling about half the collection they start to become confused. We then smell each plant one by one. The best score among my clients is properly identifying six out of the fourteen plants. But that doesn't matter; once you describe the fragrance again to each person, and then they smell the same plant, they are able to separate the different scents.

"Compare the lemon-rose to the lime geranium. Try to discern the difference and separate the fragrances," I implore. The class samples each and are able to smell the slight hint of rose scent in the lemon-rose geranium when compared to the lime. "You can really tell the difference when you know what you are smelling," says Lily. They spend the rest of the class smiling as they rub the leaves, smelling their fingers and appreciating the differences.

STAIRWAY TO RASPBERRIES

It is time to build a set of stairs in the hill that holds the raspberry (*Rubus idaeus*) bushes we planted in the Children's Garden. Tracy and I decide to construct stairs to make it easier to walk between the rows. We will also eliminate a ditch that is forming from the rain runoff created by the raised beds we built last year in the upper garden that was prone to flooding. The good news about the upper garden is that it doesn't flood as much as it used to; the bad news is that the water needs to go somewhere.

With this in mind, and leftover pressure-treated four-by-fours, we start to build the stairs. My first lesson is to teach my students how to measure and use a bubble level. I hold up the level for each child, showing how the little bubble within a tube of liquid needs to rest in the center between two thin lines to determine whether the object is level. Most are able to pick up this skill fairly quickly.

"Ellen, is it level?" I ask after setting a timber into the ground.

"Yes it is," replies Ellen, holding the level securely against the timber, pointing out that the bubble sits perfectly balanced between the two lines on the tube.

The students get a good sense of accomplishment from helping to build the stairs. We use a pickax to dig out a triangular chunk of soil to form a step. After ensuring the cut for the step is level, we measure how long each timber needs to be, one in front and two for the sides, and then cut each one with a chop saw. We use a portable drill to pre-drill the holes for the spikes that will hold the timbers together. After nailing the timbers together, we hammer rebar steel rods into the ground on the sides and front to support and stabilize them. At the end, we dump in wheelbarrows of trap rock as a base and stone dust on top to walk on. Each child has a favorite job.

Ellen likes to use the pickax. She carefully trims off the rough spots in the dirt so that the timbers will lay flat and straight. Mateo and most of the other boys like to drill. They all follow the same learning curve. I tell them to press slowly and hold the drill with both hands so it will not torque out of their grip. They all ignore this advice and hold it with one hand, and the drill spins out of control predictably.

"Wow that is really strong," says Mateo.

"Yes it is, Mateo. How do you think it is able to drill through wood so easily? Hold it with both hands and press the button gently." After a few tries Mateo masters the drill.

Measuring lengths of wood tests the children's abilities differently. I use the chore of measuring lengths with a tape measure as a way to teach simple arithmetic. A few children use it for multiplication by counting off large units like feet. No one becomes frustrated as I help them with the counting, and we get to the right place on the measuring tape.

Another skill where their abilities differ is hammering. Pre-drilling the timbers eases the task, but we still need to put spikes through two inches of undrilled wood, which is taxing even for me. Most of the children quit after they start to hit undrilled wood, though one child, Edward, is determined to hammer all of his spikes in. With each swing he becomes more determined, even though the power he is able to deliver decreases with each attempt. After smashing in two spikes, he turns the hammer over to me with sweaty pleasure. "It's your turn now, Mr. Keller."

That is how it goes the entire day as we work our way from the bottom up. The day flies by for all my charges with no one wanting to go back to class. Each wants to stay to finish the job. To me that is the best lesson that I can give them and shows me that sometimes the foremost job in the garden doesn't include plants.

JUNE CRAFT: MAKE CUTTINGS

When plants are in full growth mode it is time to make propagation cuttings to spread around your garden or give to friends and family. Some plants, such as any mint or forsythia bushes (Forsythia suspensa), can be propagated by cutting it and literally dropping the cuttings on the ground: they will always root. Other plants, however, require a little more care.

Soft tissue plants such as geraniums, chrysanthemums (Chrysanthemum), coleus (Plectranthus scutellarioides), and most herbs can be rooted simply in a container of water or growing medium such as perlite. Shrubs can also be propagated by cutting off the new succulent tips just as they are beginning to harden. The odds of success can be increased by dipping a stem into rooting hormone and then putting the end in perlite or a light soil mix. When

roots begin to form, the plant can be transferred to a
pot of soil or put directly into the ground.

CUTTING FLOWERS, EXPOSING MEMORIES

A goal of horticultural therapy is to help clients work through or at least recognize their challenges. Before you can begin to do that, particularly for clients with emotional or social issues, you must first gain your client's trust. Working in the Children's Garden at Green Chimneys, I have found that one of the easiest ways to obtain trust is to use a skill from my former profession as a consultant and be a good listener by striking up conversations during quiet tasks.

The chives have bloomed and the flowers need to be cut to preserve the bulb. The day is cloudless, windy, but very comfortable. We have ideal conditions to kneel down and snip the heads off the flowers. It doesn't matter how much of the chive flowers we cut, but to make it more challenging and precise I have the group of students I am mentoring snip them toward the top of the stem where the flower sits. This forces them to concentrate on the job rather than prune indiscriminately.

While many of the pink puff-ball-like flower heads are starting to go to seed, others are still fresh and attracting bees. Some students panic and scream when they spot these flying insects.

"Don't worry," I say calmly. "As long as you are not threatening, they will not bother you. Move away from the flowers and watch me." They retreat happily. I take their place, and with my trusty Felco clippers, enter a patch of chives filled with bees. There are a few gasps with the expectation that I will be attacked. I carefully and slowly remove the flowers with a few bees landing on my hand but without being stung. After being horrified initially, the children calm down and believe that I am some type of bee whisperer.

Following my example, all except one start working among the bees with a little trepidation but remain in control of their fears. After a short time, no one has been stung, and the onion-like smell of the stalks and flowers of the chives coats our hands. It is pleasant and soothing though pungent.

Later I am working alone with Bob. After a while sitting, he starts speaking about his Summer and the trips he will be taking with his mother and stepfather. He then starts to speak about his grandfather. "I don't ever want to meet my grandfather. He's a bad man." Bob talks about how his grandfather is an alcoholic and would beat his father, even when his father, also an alcoholic, was older. "My mom doesn't drink," he adds.

Bob talks about his family in a calm and matter-of-fact tone. He clips the flowers carefully, dropping them into a tote, and continues to tell me his story. "They could have stopped drinking if they wanted to. It's all their fault. They're bad." A tear forms in one of his eyes and he stops working.

"Bob, alcoholism is a disease that never leaves you, even if you stop drinking. Yes, perhaps they could stop drinking, but it's not easy and it's a constant battle. I'm sorry that their actions hurt you," I say.

"It doesn't matter anymore," says Bob. "They're not part of me or my Mom's life." Bob is silent, so we stop talking and finish removing the flowers from a clump of chives. Bob does such a good job I let him harvest the first of the strawberries as well as a few gooseberries as a treat. "This is a good day," he says, as I walk him back to class.

Jada, my next student, has a different reaction around the chives. She works near other students in a group that I am managing and becomes very possessive about cutting a certain number of flowers in a specific area. "These are mine!" she shouts manically. I give her a wide berth and let her cut the flowers. She does a good job, sometimes lingering and looking at the individual blooms while delicately holding them in her hand.

I later take her aside and ask why she is so possessive. "I don't know. I guess I just wanted to have my own space and do it on my own."

One of my last students, Josh, is making quick work of the job. He cuts the heads closely and quickly. He discovers the heads that have mostly gone to seed are easy to pull off the stalks. "Is it okay if I pull them rather than cut them?"

I reply yes, but he has to make sure that the flower is past and gone to seed. I demonstrate to him the difficulty in trying to pull off a live flower versus the relative ease of removing a seed pod. He nods and then says, "These smell like stink bugs." I didn't know the type of bug he is referring to, so I ask him to describe one to me. He then starts to look bothered and says that he doesn't want to. I ask why.

"They live in the country where I was born. It's not a nice place. I don't want to remember anything about it."

"Would you like to talk about this?"

"No, because if I do, I won't be able to stop, and I want to forget about ever coming from there."

Josh is now agitated. I need to change the topic. "Josh, how would you like some strawberries?" His mood starts to change. "Is there any asparagus left?"

"Yes, I think so, and there may be some gooseberries for you also."

His face brightens, so we pick up our pruners, knee pads, and tote of chive flowers and walk toward the shed to put them away. "Do you think I could have two strawberries, Mr. Keller?"

"Sure, Josh," I reply. "If you can find two ripe ones." He runs off toward the strawberry patch in front of me, forgetting the chives and thinking about the strawberries that he hopes to find.

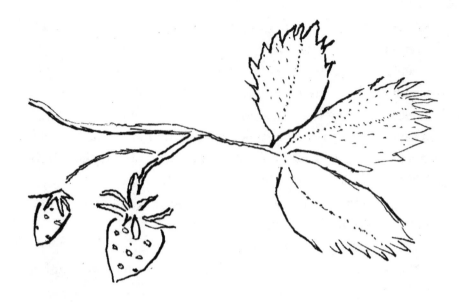

BIRDS, 0; SLUGS, 0; GRANDPARENTS, 0; CHARLOTTE, 10 AND COUNTING

I took extra pains this year to minimize the potential for carnage to my strawberry patch, attempting to anticipate every pest that could strip my plants clean of the berries we so much covet this time of year. I cleaned the beds of all detritus in early Spring to minimize fungal diseases. I sprinkled iron phosphate pellets, which act as an organic stomach poison for slugs and snails by damaging their digestive tracts, eventually causing their death. I then placed straw around the strawberry plants so that the berries would not rot on the damp soil. Finally, I encircled the bed with bird netting so that even a tiny finch or chipmunk cannot find its way into the area. The garden's fencing, gate, and slats have been repaired so a skinny Peter Rabbit or a fat woodchuck will be thwarted.

But I never considered Charlotte.

Charlotte is my trusty garden helper, coming every day to water, weed, and harvest. A favorite stop in the vegetable garden is my thriving sorrel patch. She walks over, grabs a few leaves with her tiny hands and then shoves the mass into her open jaw. A plump mouthful is worked like a good chaw of tobacco by a baseball player, but then she swallows it and often goes back for seconds.

Charlotte doesn't realize what tasty treasures are growing under the veil of netting until we find the first strawberry of the season. It is a tiny orange heirloom sample that is barely ripe but perfect in all other ways. I ask Charlotte if she wants to get it.

"Charlotte wants to eat strawberry," is her assertive reply.

And with that first but tiny offering, a little strawberry monster is born.

Every day Charlotte insists that we need to check the garden at least twice to see if any new berries have ripened. She is a much better berry spotter than I, as I need to bend down and look through the leaves and I miss a lot of fruit. Charlotte, on the other hand, easily looks through the stems and leaves with the precision of a trained berry picker or a young Supergirl with X-ray vision.

"Pampi, strawberry there," she says pointing out her next snack.

"Where Charlotte? I can't see it?"

"There, Pampi," she replies pointing her right index finger toward the soon to be grabbed and ingested fruit.

And she is always right. Behind the leaves is a nice red strawberry.

While Charlotte often helps me with harvests, when it comes to strawberries, she is more apt to help herself. Her tiny hands can fit under the netting in ways a chipmunk cannot. And the tiniest berries are extracted through the netting by her delicate little fingers. She misses nothing in the strawberry patch. These little harvests are popped into her mouth quickly, while larger specimens have a slightly greater chance of being shared with Juana or myself, if we can get a bite in before Charlotte clamps her teeth on the remaining morsel.

SUMMER SOLSTICE SUPPER

For the Summer solstice I do something special for my clients at Ann's Place and prepare a nice dinner that is locally sourced. After all, this is in sync with many cultures that celebrate the end of darkness and hunger and the beginning of Summer abundance.

Gathering the makings for this dinner is half the fun. I visit surrounding farm stands as well as plan out my own home harvests so I have enough fresh food to prepare for the group. The weather cooperates with a temperate and clear day. All my clients have arrived.

We gather as a group on the veranda at Ann's Place that overlooks the backyard. A nearby condominium complex is shielded from view by a thick curtain of trees and Japanese barberry (*Berberis thunbergii*) bushes. To our left, the daffodils (*Narcissus*) are spent for the season and replaced by swaths of native ferns (*Tracheophyta*). The fescue (*Festuca*) lawn has been cut recently. Clients are chatting among themselves, beverage in hand. The insects are in abeyance.

I start with a reading from *Herb Gardening in Five Seasons*, by Adelma Simmons, who used to run the Caprilands Herb Farm in nearby Coventry, Connecticut. It speaks of the party we are having.

We have a celebration for midsummer . . . the time of the Summer solstice, the longest days of the year. . . . Wheels to represent the sun were wrapped with straw and smeared with pitch, lighted and rolled down hill toward water, this to insure good crops for the year. Cattle were driven through the fire to protect them from sickness and bewitching. Young couples jumped over the flames, the higher they leaped, the taller their crops would grow.

With this and some observations by the group of how our gardens have changed in the last few months, we stroll the grounds. Our walk begins at the herb garden, and I start by giving everyone a tiny piece of stevia (*Stevia rebaudiana*). "Put it on your tongue and just let it sit," I tell the group, feeling like a Christian minister dispensing communion wafers.

"Wow, that is really sweet!"

Summer Solstice Menu

Salad red butternut, slow bolt, and tango lettuce (*Lactuca sativa*); sorrel (*Rumex acetosa*); purslane (*Portulaca oleracea*); garlic (*Allium sativum*) scapes; radishes (*Raphanus sativus*); snow peas (*Pisum sativum* var. *saccharatum*)

Potato (*Solanum tuberosum*) **baguettes**

Chevre, Gruyere, Farmstead cheeses

Garlic scape pesto & pasta

Smoked trout and breast of chicken

Blueberries (*Vaccinium corymbosum*)

Strawberries (*Fragaria ×ananassa*)

Strawberry-rhubarb (*Rheum rhabarbarum*) **pie**

"That's incredible."

"What did you call this plant?"

"Now try to discern the nuances between the mints. They are quite distinct," I say as I point to the fifteen different ones we have lining the walk. With that, everyone starts to scratch and sniff all the plants, slowly at first and then more quickly as they capture as much scent as possible. The group lingers, enveloped with fragrance. We continue our walk. My guests are full of questions.

"I have this one in my backyard, what is it?" Garlic mustard (*Alliaria petiolata*).

"Is this poison ivy (*Toxicodendron radicans*)?" No, it is Jack-in-the-pulpit (*Arisaema triphyllum*).

"What are these dead-looking leaves?" They are daffodils. "We don't remove them until they totally die," I explain. "Should be in a couple of weeks."

"What is this cute purple flower?" I have no idea.

Clients start to spread out in the back garden. Some linger on benches looking at the new sculptures that were installed last week. Others continue to test my plant-identification abilities.

"That is Oriental bittersweet (*Celastrus orbiculatus*). If you have it in your yard, you want to remove it.

"This is a viburnum (*Viburnum*); I'm not sure which cultivar.

"These are witch hazels (*Hamamelis virginiana*). This particular species has a wonderful, delicate little yellow flower that blooms in November."

My clients are enjoying the walk, quiet in their thoughts. I pass a sample of Queen Anne's lace (*Daucus carota*) down the line of clients, telling them to smell the root, and I can see that everyone is peaceful and mindful of the garden at Ann's Place. Some follow me around the path, others take up residence on one of the many benches lining the walkway. The tour is over.

I tell my lingering clients to join me in ten minutes for a meal on the veranda. Everything is staged in the kitchen; I need to set it out and hope that the menu choice is diverse enough to please everyone.

A few clients return with me to the building and help me set out the food, and soon we all congregate on the veranda. I inquire if anyone would like wine served. Most hands shoot up, making me happy that I brought three bottles of white wine from a local vineyard. I then read a short passage from *The Rural Life* by Verlyn Klinkenborg.

But as far as I can tell, no one's eating the slugs. We try not to... The garden is flecked with them in the early morning and after I've tossed a few of them into the nettle patch, the revulsion they cause dies away—until one turns up on the salad plate.

"Bon appétit!"

Cries of "gross" and "yuck" arise with nervous laughter. The unintended consequences of eating food that is organic and fresh are often overlooked. The evening and meal pass quickly as conversation fills the veranda with little care or attention to time. Music accompanies the quiet sound of birds and insects in the background. We exchange recipes and memories of the meals and gardens of our youth with every mouthful of food. Worries are gone as everyone is happy and content with the meal. The wine is gone. I bring out dessert, coffee, and tea. No one is in a hurry. We linger until darkness begins to descend. Reluctantly we know it is time to go, as the chirping of birds fades and bats arrive to feast on insects swarming overhead.

JUNE OUTING: TAKE A HIKE

With vegetation in full bloom, a walk anywhere can reveal treasures. In your yard, new plants seeded by animals or wind have emerged. In a nearby park or woods, a flower that you may have never noticed comes into view.

The leaf litter of Winter has become humus, feeding the trees and other flora. The soil is alive with not only new growth but scents and textures that have been missed, or even long since forgotten. Sounds are more muffled as growing vegetation mutes noises. It is time to take in the new season with all of your senses.

OLD PERENNIALS, NEW SPROUTS

The garden is always changing, this year more than usual. The past Winter brought shocks of hot and cold that have taken their toll on the butterfly bush (*Buddleia davidii*), rose, and hydrangea (*Hydrangea*) bushes, forcing either their removal or extreme cutting back to their roots. Juana's fig tree (*Ficus carica*) is pushing just a few green shoots; I will be surprised if any figs greet us this year.

The same is true with my clients at Ann's Place, given their struggles and diagnoses. Some come back every season. Others do not. With every session it is always a surprise to find who, how many, and the condition of those who show up to pot plants, make sachets, or participate in any other of my activities. Much like facing reality with my decade-old bushes, I feel a particular sadness and melancholy when a long-time client is unable to attend my classes. This is different from my happiness when clients choose not to attend as the normalcy and recovery from cancer make my class superfluous. But the absence of others are harder to take. And there is one client in particular.

Beth started to attend my class years ago. Initially she was very quiet but soon started to correct me when I made a misstatement.

"No Erik, that is not a raspberry but rather a wineberry (*Rubus phoenicolasius*). You can tell by the smaller thorns and the berry's shape.

"I think you mean an iris (*Iris*) rather than a daylily (*Hemerocallis*).

"Lemon balm (*Melissa officinalis*) is part of the mint family. Just check the stem."

In a prior life I would have become upset over such corrections, but now I realize that I still have much to learn about gardening and being corrected is one of the best things that can help increase my knowledge.

As Beth and I start to converse more, a playful banter emerges between us. I discover that she has a bachelor's degree in horticulture and has worked on farms and gardens all her life. I should have noticed her strong and rough hands, indicating a life of outdoor labor, in addition to her knowledgeable comments. Unlike many of my other charges, she plays in the soil like my granddaughter, without any regard of messiness or dirtying her hands or clothes. Her workspace is always the most soiled. We always need to swap out the table paper after a potting up exercise with her.

But a few months ago Beth stopped attending as her health took a downturn, severely limiting her mobility and preventing her from getting to my class. This was hard to take. Whenever she joined our class on walks, she was always reaching out and grabbing an errant weed or picking a pretty flower.

"You really need to get rid of this mugwort (*Artemisia vulgaris*), Erik. It's quite invasive."

"I know, Beth, it's on my list."

I miss having this helpful thorn by my side. I phone her, offering to make a house visit with a flat of tomato and pepper (*Capsicum annuum*) plants so she and a friend can plant up her garden.

"Oh that would be wonderful. I haven't had time to start anything this year."

Entering her home, which is an old, battered white trailer with green trim, Juana and I see a crowded space with decades of memories spilling off her shelves. Beth greets us with a tired smile and a big hug. Over the next hour she is making a mess on her kitchen table, potting up plants and loving every minute of it. Upon leaving, Beth gives Juana a tiny ceramic statue as thanks for our visit.

I invite her to my next class in a week but know inside that she will not come; I am right. At that session, we identify mints and scented geraniums. A first-time client, much younger, starts to pepper me with questions.

"You asked us our favorite smell. What's yours?"

"Lilac, but when my wife is baking, apple pie."

"Why do the mints smell different?" I tell her I thought it was the chemistry of each plant but I really don't know.

"How did scented geraniums come about?" I tell her I thought it was most likely through selective breeding, but again I didn't know for sure.

While Beth is no longer in attendance and I will never see her again, a new thorn appears to be taking her place.

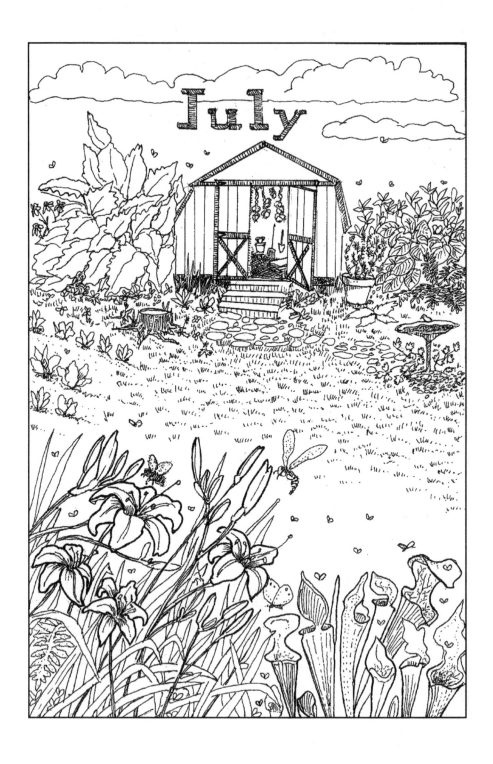

JULY: HOT, HOT, HOT

July is the month of heat, homemade ice cream, and the desire to remain cool. It is an ironic time, as the weather and gardens have flipped into high gear after a long stasis. The warm evenings find fireflies illuminating the background for all the nocturnal creatures. Torrential rains are both common and fleeting, as the heat of the day helps to release accumulated moisture in a loud and boisterous thunderstorm that comes and goes with the flick of an eye.

Summer vegetables—peppers (Capsicum annuum), tomatoes (Solanum lycopersicum), and beans (Phaseolus vulgaris)—come into their own. Depending upon moisture, the grounds will look lush with growth or parched with thirst. Strawberries (Fragaria ×ananassa) have already left most gardens but have been replaced with blueberries (Vaccinium corymbosum), wineberries (Rubus phoenicolasius), and raspberries (Rubus idaeus). There is much to look at and eat.

GETTING THE GARLIC

It has become more challenging to determine when certain crops should be planted and picked. I took a chance this year with my tomatoes, putting them in the garden two weeks before Memorial Day. I was rewarded, for once, with hot weather that caused them to double in size weekly. They are over five feet high in cages that are full of flowers and tiny tomatoes.

Garlic (*Allium sativum*) is easier to time, as it is planted in Fall before the frost and pulled in mid to late July, or even August. Like leeks (*Allium porrum*), garlic is a crop with a long gestation and big rewards that can't be seen until harvest. Planting garlic cloves in the cool of Fall is one of the last acts of planting for the season. In early to mid November you observe that the teeth are sprouting, but the cold stops their progress and snow covers them until Spring.

By April, garlic leaves poke through the straw as they emerge toward the sun. Unlike other years, I had hard neck scapes ready to cut and sauté last month. Typically, that means that the bulbs will be ready to harvest in a few weeks, early by past years. Each day as I tour the garden, I look for signs of readiness. Tips going brown, bottom leaves dying, a small amount of wilt in the plant. And today the trifecta of signs all line up, so Charlotte and I decide it is harvest time.

I leave the straw on the garlic bed rather than remove it. The straw keeps the soil moist and minimizes the need to water or weed. Charlotte takes the first tug of a garlic stalk with her little hands attempting to liberate it from the soil. "This is hard, Pampi."

We both hear a slow and steady tear as the roots free themselves from the soil. Out pops a fragrant and large garlic bulb. "We did it!" she shouts. We pull the other bulbs in sequence. Charlotte enjoys pulling and lining them up in groups of ten so we can count how many we harvest. We finish with thirteen piles, 130 heads in all.

I planted many garlic cloves last year, as I was unsure how well the crop would do given the prior year's harvest, which consisted of a few smaller bulbs. Each tug shows us, however, that regardless of Winter conditions, the garlic came through very well.

Rows of garlic are drying on my greenhouse wire racks, shaded with newspaper so they will not burn. The fan in the greenhouse will keep the air moving and dry. In prior years, I have put them in the shed in the back, but the greenhouse, now with its shade cloth on, should do the trick. My greenhouse is now full of the sweet-and-sour scent of garlic as the fan spins, keeping the temperature cool while the garlic dries, waiting to be braided.

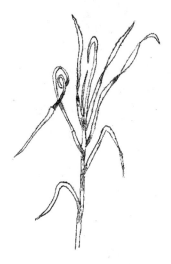

GROWING WITH CLIENTS

Recent classes at Ann's Place have taken my students to the herb gardens to learn how to identify each herb by sight and smell. They touch and caress different plants, asking questions and making mental notes.

It is this type of discovery that I hope my clients will experience with me. With each class I wind up throwing lots of different "bait" out to see what resonates best. During last week's class I played a Gloria Estefan CD, because I thought her music was perfect for the hot and sultry weather we were having. And I was right.

"That music is wonderful," said one client. "I feel like we are in Cuba. Is that Gloria Estefan?"

On the other hand, the soundtrack for "Little Shop of Horrors" was not well received when we were working with carnivorous plants, so it quickly came off the CD player.

When clients sit down with each other, I want them to lose themselves in the moment. And they often do with banter and a sense of sharing. This type of comfortable chatting permeates the sessions, with everyone looking to help each other.

I have realized that when I offer them plant samples at the close of class, it is a mark of a successful session when my clients do their best to avoid becoming like crazed Walmart shoppers on Black Friday.

"Does anyone want this last plant?" asks one client, sheepishly hoping that the answer will be no. Some do their best to slyly corral the specimens they want by diversion, while others make a quick plunging grab, much as would a hovering pelican diving for a fishy meal.

But even these exercises are done with the best intentions, as when we finish potting up everyone helps clean up and admires their neighbors' creations. No one is unhappy with their choices, in the same way that all of our children are beautiful. They then leave the basement, arms full of pots and herbs, happy, with soil under their nails and smiles on their faces.

FIRST BITE

The raspberries and wineberries have arrived. It is easy to confuse the two, with their similar looking and tasting fruits. Raspberry bushes are distinguished by their long distinctive thorns on smooth vines, while wineberries have somewhat fuzzy vines with more closely spaced and shorter thorns. The differences matter little to Juana and Charlotte as both want to harvest berries: They see fruit ready to eat. Unfortunately, this year the berries have taken up residence on the back hill surrounded by poison ivy (*Toxicodendron radicans*) and other weeds that are perilous to walk though. Compounding the difficulty is the fact that some of the bushes thick with fruit have grown in and near piles of brush containing old rose (*Rosa*) stems and other prickly branches.

We should approach this wearing long pants and gloves, but only I have gloves. We are lucky that we can get shoes on Charlotte. She has taken to running around the backyard unshod as would any of the animals that snack on our garden.

I open the gate, approaching the bushes with pruners, pointing out and removing poison ivy and dropping it out of the way. I move thorny branches to the side and start to clear a path so we can safely walk though.

We start harvesting berries with Juana and I placing them into our baskets and Charlotte into her mouth. Charlotte is happy and sated as dark pink juice begins to coat her lips and a small trickle runs down her face. Her fingers are dark from the picking. All of a sudden Charlotte starts to scream. I look about and see a tiny wasp attached to her ankle. I swat it away but the damage has been done.

Charlotte has received her first sting, or more accurately, bite. She attempts to be brave, but the tears start running down her cheek. I quickly go over to our patch of jewelweed (*Impatiens capensis*) and pull some leaves while Juana consoles Charlotte. I pick Charlotte up, cradling her in my arms, while Juana makes a poultice from the leaves and applies it to the bite. In a few minutes the swelling in her ankle abates and she stops crying. She must have accidentally stepped on a nest or bothered the wasp as it was foraging. It was a very tiny wasp, but for Charlotte it was huge. We return to the house to rest. Sitting down, she draws a picture of what happened to show her mother and father. It is not to scale; the wasp is the size of a bird attached to her ankle. A few tears continue to line her cheeks.

After Charlotte calms down, we return to the woods and are extra careful picking berries. Soon our baskets are full. We take these berries as well as the blueberries that we have just harvested and wash them for lunch. Charlotte enjoys a large bowl of mixed berries with whipped cream. Her welt from the bite is now a bit itchy underneath a Band-Aid, but she has a smile on her face: A second helping is about to be served.

JULY CRAFT: COLLECT PLANTS TO PRESS

Flowers are now blooming en masse and it is time to preserve some for colder and darker days. Collecting and pressing flowers is simple and can be done throughout Summer. To start, a flower press is needed. A flower press can be as simple as a large book. Or, many people build or buy a more complex, wooden-framed device having cardboard and paper layers to compress with thumbscrews.

The task of pressing flowers is fairly simple though several rules should be followed: 1) Plants to press should not be wet, 2) plants with fat centers or parts should be avoided, and 3) plants should be put into paper sleeves that are folded on each other between the cardboard layers or pages of a book. It takes between three and six weeks for the plants to dry before they are ready to be used for a variety of projects.

BUNNIES AND SLUGS AND BUGS, OH MY!

My horticultural-therapy classes are usually planned well in advance, but sometimes I need to scramble. Today thunderstorms are expected for the entire day, so working in the garden or greenhouse is not possible. I need to come up with an alternative that will hold interest in a small windowless classroom, a depressing space to teach teenage girls languishing in a detention facility.

I put on my rain jacket and go outside trying to figure out what I can collect that will interest the girls. I don't want to disappoint, as I have been gaining their confidence over the past few months; they are starting to really enjoy gardening and working with plants. After a lap around my house, an idea comes to me and I start gathering materials and supplies.

Later that day, I am crammed into a small room with six girls, all dressed in white and black sweats, the standard detention-facility garb. They fidget, unhappy that they can't go outside and bothered that we are sitting in a circle with a couple of boxes in the center and one behind me.

"I am sorry that we can't go outside," I say. "But it is too dangerous given the thunder and lightning." Almost on cue a large rumbling noise penetrates our bunker-like room. "So today, we are going to have a lesson on garden pests."

With that I remove a few coleus (*Plectranthus scutellarioides*) leaves from a box and pass them and a few magnifying glasses around the circle. I ask the girls to tell me what they see.

"I see some white dots," says Elise.

"I think they have legs. That's gross," says Kate.

The girls play with the magnifying glasses, as half of them have never used one.

"This is a white fly. A really bad pest. If your plant gets infested, it is better sometimes to get rid of the plant than try to cure it," I say. "If you do want to get rid of the flies, there are different techniques." I then describe the ways to rid the plant of these pests including spraying them with insecticidal soap.

I pull out the next sample, a bean leaf that looks like a skeleton. There are a few bugs on its underside.

"These are ladybugs," says Sarah. "Though their color is wrong." The other girls start nodding their heads.

"Well, I have a couple of ladybugs in this package," I say, pulling out a plastic bag. The girls look and notice a difference.

"Also, this class is about garden pests. Ladybugs are garden helpers that eat aphids and other bugs that do damage to plants," I explain. "These are Mexican bean beetles, which is another really bad pest. I let them get out of control and they are ruining all my beans. Look at both carefully."

The girls pass the samples around examining the differences. The biggest difference is color. The ladybug is a darker red while the bean beetle is an orange-brown. The bean beetle is also bigger than a ladybug.

The girls are enjoying the Nature show and tell. I bring out the next pest.

"Gross."

"Disgusting!"

"Yuck."

There is universal repulsion to the two slugs that ooze their way over a piece of cardboard. I have a very large leopard slug that has black spots on a dark green body and a tinier yellow one that appears almost fluorescent. They both leave a slime trail as they move forward.

Interest in these gastropods is minimal, as is the discussion I have about the damage they do and how to keep them in check in gardens. I return them to my bag.

"Okay, girls, I have saved the worst predator of the garden for last," I say. "You don't want any of these to go into your garden. They are deadly to plants." And with that, I pull out our pet rabbit, Pooh, from a box behind me.

"Oh my god, it's so cute," says Elise.

"Can I hold it?" asks Nia.

"Me too!" chime the others. I pass Pooh around and tell the girls about how damaging mammals are in the garden. "Peter the rabbit is not so nice if you are Mr. McGregor," I say. But my words fall on deaf ears as the girls are all smiles and happy that a cute bunny has brightened their rainy day.

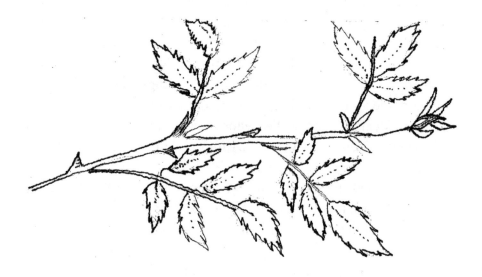

SMELLING THE ROSES, REMEMBERING MOTHER

My mother's garden on Long Island continues to please her and amaze her neighbors. After my father's death from cancer, my mother has become much more comfortable in her yard. She is looking after it with attention and pride. The last time I checked in on my mother, her sister was visiting from Florida and it was time to trim the roses. A few months earlier my mother didn't realize she had a rose bush, but it was there, hidden in plain sight.

After we had rehabilitated the two front beds of the house mid Spring, we went to the backyard and saw an out-of-control Oriental bittersweet (*Celastrus orbiculatus*). As I started to pull it out I realized that a rose bush and a Japanese maple (*Acer palmatum*) were covered by the choking leaves and vine.

"Mom, do you know you have a rose bush in the back?"

"What rose bush?"

After I pointed it out, she had no idea how the rose got there. But I had an idea.

When we were young, my father installed a split-rail fence around our corner-situated property and planted a rose bush between each set of posts. In the early years, they bloomed expansively with buckets of flowers covering the top rails. They were planted in colored sequence—yellow, red, white, pink—up the side street and around the front. My mother used to go out to smell the roses and look with contentment at her flowering property line. But years of children trampling and lawn mowers not respecting them led to their gradual and inevitable demise, so that decades later only a few specimens survived. (These survivors were a blessing for me, as I used to clip their flowers and bring a bouquet to my future mother-in-law while I was courting my wife.)

My father eventually took down the fence, and I believe he took the single remaining rose bush and planted it in the backyard without telling anyone. More than a decade later, my mother and I found it. I cut down and removed the bittersweet. The maple I was able to dig out with a nice ball of soil around its roots. My mother decided to plant it near the corner of the house, so we excavated a hole and added lots of manure and compost.

That was a few months ago, and since then the roses have been plentiful and the unfettered bush has tripled in size. Now it is time to deadhead the roses.

With my aunt Nancy watching, I give my mother a pair of pruners, and she is able to squeeze them with her weak, arthritic hands. This is an amazing feat for her. A few years ago she would not take care of a plastic plant; now she is enthusiastically and carefully trimming off the dead branches and buds of a rose bush that was first planted on our property in the 1960s—more than forty years ago. She starts on one side of the bush clipping away randomly, letting the dead branches and buds drop to the ground. We reminisce about the house's old rose bushes and those at her mother's house. She uses her cane to push the cuttings into a pile, making it easy for me to rake up everything and cart it away. I take the pruner from her to remove the spent buds she cannot reach. She directs me on what to cut and where. "You missed that one in the back. . . . Not so much from the front. . . . Don't forget that one."

After we finish we sit down in the backyard with glasses of iced tea. I ask my mother and Nancy about their mother and if she was an avid gardener. "Oh yes," says Nancy. "Mother had a wonderful garden."

"We used to make dolls out of hollyhocks (*Alcea*)," adds my mother.

The sisters start to reminisce about their mother's garden. There was a line of lilies (*Lilium*) near the side of their childhood home, along with white, purple, yellow, and pale violet irises (*Iris*). Nancy's favorite flower in the garden was the peony (*Paeonia*). My mother loved the pink and purple lilacs (*Syringa vulgaris*) that bloomed in her mother's backyard.

In the back of the house there was a rock garden fronting large patches of Oriental poppies (*Papaver orientale*) where my aunt and mother as children played dress up with their mother's old clothing. They argue over who played the princess most often. They vividly describe the different colors and types of flowers that were around the rock garden, and how they would roll down the hill at their uncle Bill's farm where they spent many Summer vacations.

They laugh and exchange playful stories about their childhood. I sit back taking sips of my tea to watch how having just a little garden has changed my mother. She now enjoys going outside to water and deadhead her flowers. It makes her feel good, especially when the neighbors notice and compliment her on how nice everything looks in her yard. And for me it's gratifying, as I listen to stories about her youth and my grandmother that I would never have heard otherwise.

JULY OUTING: PICK BERRIES

There is never a better time to go berry picking than in the heat of July, which offers an embarrassment of *wild blueberries (*Vaccinium angustifolium*), gooseberries (*Ribes uva-crispa*), raspberries, wineberries, and at the end of the month, blackberries (*Rubus fruticosus*). If there are weedy samples of these Summer treats nearby your home, all the better, as an early stroll can also double as fruit collection for the morning's breakfast.*

If you don't have these bushes on your property or along the roadside, don't be deterred, as there are many farms where you can pick your own. Children in particular love these destinations, because they often carry away more berries in their tummies than in baskets. There is nothing more delicious than fresh, fully ripened berries just off the vine. Once you sample this ambrosia, you are hooked.

THE FUNGUS AMONG US

Though July is supposed to be hot, Mother Nature doesn't always deliver. The wet, cool weather we have been having in the Northeast is the perfect catalyst for fungal spores. And tomatoes are among the most vulnerable to this circumstance.

In the Children's Garden, the entire tomato patch is infested with fusarium wilt. It is threatening to wipe out our tomatoes, which are essential for Summer Salsa, a big favorite. And while best practices say that you should rip out the plants, we can't do that just yet. So we do the next best thing: containment and clean-up.

As I start the job of clipping desiccated branches from the infected plants, two students and their teacher come to the garden to look around. They look at me, wondering what I am doing. I motion for them to come over.

"What do you see about this plant that doesn't look right?" I ask.

"Some leaves have spots," says one. "There is gross stuff over there," says the other, pointing toward a bunch of shriveled, brown leaves.

I cut a couple of branches and explain to them the pathology and progression of the fungus, how it starts and then grows and then kills the branches of the plant that it infects. I will be repeating this explanation most of the day to others.

My first student, Susan, seems shy at first, but by the time we get out of the school building and into the garden she is active and animated. I try to speak quietly with all the children before we get into the garden, to gauge their mental and emotional states so that we can select the best chore for our time together.

Susan and I sit down and review all the different things we will need to do during our hour together. Removing wilt from tomato plants requires different skills and coordination of cognitive abilities. The student needs to identify which stems need cutting, navigate through a plant with a pruning tool, and then cut it close to the stem without damaging the larger plant (or a finger).

The student must also remove all diseased leaves and place them in a bucket and clean the surrounding grounds of fallen-off leaves while trying not to brush the infected leaves against healthy ones. After each plant is groomed, the clippers then need to be sterilized in a bleach or alcohol solution and the leaves disposed of so that they do not come into contact with other plants or soil in the garden. Lots of sequencing needs to occur to get it all right.

Susan appears interested and eager to work on the task at hand. The key thing about any job in the garden is that it should stimulate and calm a student. In this case, Susan asks question after question about gardening and Nature. We soon get to the point of working side-by-side, trimming the visibly infected leaves off the plants.

"How do tomatoes form? What is pollination? How does the fungus kill the plant? Have you ever traveled to . . . ?" With each question we stop our work and sometimes go to a different part of the garden to answer her questions.

We maintain an ongoing banter during our time together that tests my limits of introductory botany. Susan never tires of the interaction and before we both know it, it is time to clean up, get some snacks from the garden and return to class.

A TEDDY BECOMES A GRIZZLY

In the garden, one of the more pleasant experiences is the sprouting of an opportunistic crop or plant. For instance, this year an ornamental squash (*Cucurbita*) started in my vegetable raised bed where I planted Swiss chard (*Beta vulgaris* subsp. *vulgaris*) in Spring. Crawling up the side of my greenhouse, it has delivered fifteen squashes with at least another six on the way in the next few days. This year's opportunistic plant in the Children's Garden at Green Chimneys is not squash but sunflowers (*Helianthus annuus*).

Three years ago, we planted three different types of sunflowers: *Helianthus annuus* 'Moulin Rouge' (all red), *H. giganteus* subsp. *alienus* (big, tall, and yellow), and *H. annuus* 'Ring of Fire' (red in the center, yellow on the edges). Since then we have not planted a single sunflower, but each year we keep getting more and more sunflowers in the garden. This year they are as thick as chickweed (*Stellaria media*) and we need to remove a lot more than we would like to.

But the interesting thing about these sunflowers is that few show any resemblance to their forbears. We have many different shades and configurations of red and yellow sunflowers in the garden, because they have been cross pollinated with different cultivars for three years running. So a wild variety of sunflowers has bloomed with different heights, colors, and flower configurations.

We have a couple of sunflowers in the garden that are nearly ten feet high, with a single defiant spike daring the squirrels to climb up and eat the tasty seeds. Others have formed big clumps with small, but tall flowers.

But perhaps the strangest was a mutant *Helianthus annuus* 'Teddy Bear' that appeared a few weeks ago. At the top of one of the large clumps, about eight feet in the air, was a teddy bear sunflower blossom about the size of a small seedless watermelon. Teddy bear sunflowers grow to a maximum height of two feet, with a bright yellow, pom-pom like flower. This is not your typical teddy bear: it's a grizzly.

"This sunflower must be the result of a giganteus cross pollinating with a teddy bear that was planted in the barrels down by the administration building," says Tracy. The administration building is about half a mile away. "It's pretty cool looking." Tracy and I agree to try and save the seed of this big flower so that we can see what its offspring will look like next year.

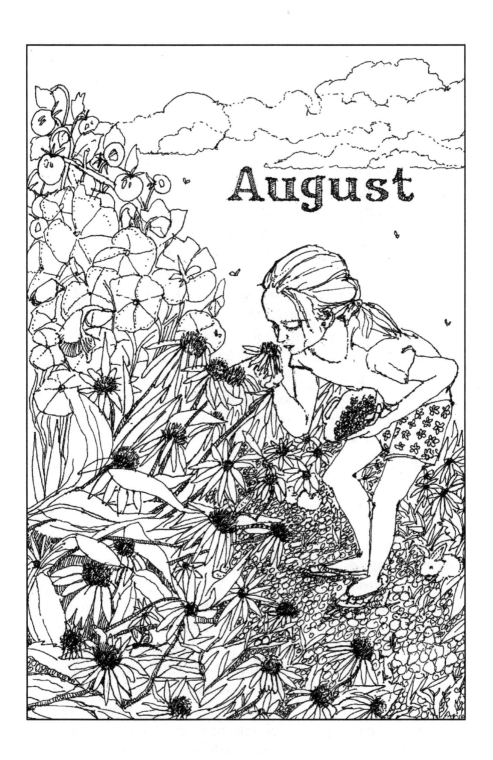

August

AUGUST: SUMMER BOUNTY

The dog days of Summer arrive in August, when the potential for unrelenting heat, afternoon thunderstorms, and extreme weather define each day. It is the hot counterpart to February, when the cold weather and cabin fever begins to wear on even the most stoic.

Favorite Summer crops such as corn (Zea mays) and watermelon (Citrullus lanatus) are harvested locally. In the North, the lakes and oceans have warmed so even the timid will take a dip into their refreshing waters. Change is in the air, where the vibrant green of Spring leaves has given way to a duller and deeper green that anticipates Fall. But such thoughts are discarded in deference to outdoor picnics and long evening walks in the presence of countless winged insects.

THE OLD BAMBOO

I have a pretty packed day today in the Children's Garden: eight sessions with eleven students between 8 a.m. and 3 p.m. Though Tracy believes I am foolhardy to agree to such a schedule, I have a good reason: I rarely ever teach all the sessions. Between absences, doctor appointments, special events, and other interruptions, someone is always dropping out. So as is typical, I find myself with some time on my hands today, and I don't feel like weeding as I had spent yesterday doing that in my home garden. Next to the barn I spot a pile of bamboo (*Bambusa vulgaris*) that Tracy ordered to build squash (*Cucurbita*) trellises and frames to hold netting for the corn. A few scraps are piled on the side. I pick one up and for some reason wonder if I can craft a flute from it.

I retract the saw from my Swiss Army knife and remove one end of the bamboo so that the stick is about a foot long with one end open and the other plugged. I brush off the cut end of splinters against the ground and open the knife's awl. I pick a random spot near the plugged end of the bamboo and start to apply pressure. By twisting the awl back and forth, a hole starts to form. Soon I have an opening that is large enough to puff across.

I put on my best flutist face and blow. Nothing. Perhaps a few fingering holes will help. After I bore in a few holes I take another shot at it. Nothing. As I have no idea what I am doing, I'm not too bothered and I keep creating more holes. I am just killing time. I then look up.

One of the boys in Tracy's class has silently walked over, staring at me and my "flute."

"What are you doing?" asks Ted.

"I'm attempting to make a flute."

"Does it work?"

"Let's see."

I then give the flute my biggest puff and best sour-lemon face. Out of the end a loud, ear-splitting noise emerges. I have built a flute. Sort of. I then plug the far end with my finger and a different sound emerges.

"That is so cool," says Ted. "Can I make one?"

The other boys in Tracy's class now saunter over to my patch of the garden and are also interested. "How about me? And me?" say two other boys. I look over to Tracy and she shrugs her shoulders, resigned to the spontaneous mutiny. I tell the boys that they can all make a flute but we will have to do it one at a time, as I have only one knife and must work closely with each to ensure safety.

"Guys, pick a piece of bamboo. But think about what you want because the larger the piece of bamboo you choose, the lower the sound will be for the flute you make and the harder you will have to blow to get a noise out of it."

Ted asks, "Why is that?" I then explain the physics of sound and why some noises have a high pitch while others do not. I explain the principle of how a flute works to the group. I teach each how to use a knife safely while holding their hands and the knife to protect them from injury. By the end of class everyone has a flute in hand and a smile on their face. No one cares about the quality of the flute's sound, but each is able to get a tweet out of their homemade instrument.

After they leave I apologize to Tracy for hijacking her class. "Oh no," she protests. "What you did was great. You were teaching them to be careful, giving them physics and music lessons at the same time. It was wonderful. Anyway, there was lots of male bonding going on—you had a knife and I can't compete with that. So why try?"

I thank Tracy for her understanding and look at the pile of bamboo next to the table. I pick out another piece for myself and plan to have another go at it during the week. Perhaps I will be able to make something that humans, rather than just dogs, can appreciate.

AUGUST CRAFT: SEED FALL GREENS WINDOW BOXES

To many it seems counter-intuitive to plant seeds in late Summer. But such sowings can bring a surprising plethora of Fall greens, radishes (Raphanus sativus), and carrots (Daucus carota subsp. sativus) that can last through the New Year. There are many ways to approach this activity. But the key is to start seeds no later than the last two weeks of August.

Starting seeds in August gives them the warmth and sunlight to grow quickly before the shortening days and cooler temperatures of Fall slow their progress. Window boxes can be moved in and around in accordance with the weather for protection and maximizing growth. Small protective hoop houses can be built to protect a crop against the weather. And with each box comes renewable, delicious salad makings that can last through the rest of the year.

BLOWING (AWAY) YOUR OWN HORN (WORM)

One of Nature's paradoxes is the inherent beauty of some things that are very harmful. Wild white berries on shrubs or trees should rarely (if ever) be eaten. The lush tropical-like leaves of New England poison ivy (*Toxicodendron radicans*) should never be touched. Never look directly into the sun during an eclipse.

Looking through the tomatoes (*Solanum lycopersicum*) in my garden I notice that the top leaves are all gone. Too high for the groundhog, whose population I presume I have eliminated based on the lack of recent damage, I ask myself, "What can it be?" Looking more closely, I discover tiny brown mounds on the lower leaves. It looks like insect feces but I don't see a bug.

As I finger through the plants I nearly touch this long, brightly colored caterpillar. It is beautiful, having a neon green body with white and yellow stripes and a series of dots on the side that look like eyes. But what is it? I show it to my wife, who quickly peruses one of our many bug books and identifies it as a tomato hornworm, which is one of the few bugs that will eat tomato leaves.

Upon reading up on these bugs I quickly determine that they are not my friends as they can devour a tomato plant overnight. After showing this creature to my wife and daughter, I trash it (literally), sending it into its afterlife. Confident, based on my experience that there is never just one pest in the garden, I go back to look for siblings and I find a few. That's the bad news.

The good news is that they are all carrying dozens of braconid parasitoid wasp larvae. Excited, I bring one to show my horrified daughter and wife. "That is so gross," says Katie. "I'm getting nauseous." Juana reacts similarly, not wanting to see the hornworm and its passengers that look like grains of rice hanging perpendicularly on the worm's body. "Get that out of my house!" she exclaims.

I comply, retiring the worm and its parasites to a patch of ground. This tomato hornworm is a host for the wasp larvae, which will kill the worm eventually and then hatch, forming a natural, native colony that will keep future hornworms in check.

I later remember these worms in the Children's Garden as we remove tomato stalks infected with bacterial speck. Removing leaves and branches with one of my students, I notice that the top of one tomato plant is missing all its leaves just like my tomato plants at home. And sure enough, beneath the missing leaves is a tomato hornworm full of parasitoid wasp larvae.

"That is so cool!" says Beth, who is helping me prune the plants. She has been withdrawn today and this new discovery perks her right up. Tracy is nearby with a class collecting tomatoes to make her homemade salsa. I bring it over to her. Never one to waste a garden pest, Tracy sits down and gives her class and my student a quick lesson on tomato hornworms, natural insect controls, and the circle of life for the parasitoid wasp. "It's kind of like Alien vs. Predator," says Tracy, "except that it's for real." I find a few more pairings, which I give to Tracy, who is now a tomato hornworm guru to the students. The kids love it.

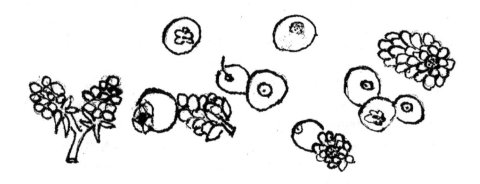

THEY BELONG IN MY TUMMY!

What makes August my favorite month in the garden is not the abundance of the crops I am harvesting, but rather the passion with which Charlotte enjoys them. When adults sink their teeth into a perfectly ripe plum (*Prunus domestica*), they usually take great care to handle the fruit, biting it carefully so all its sweet juices drip into their mouths. Not Charlotte. She grips the fruit with an intensity akin to that of a lion dispatching a wildebeest, subsequently sinking her teeth into it for a quick and efficient kill.

Juice sprays in all directions and soon her arms are coated thick with rivulets of liquid; her face is covered with pieces of her prey, suspended near her mouth. But unlike the lion she is not sated with a single kill: she wants more and could eat a half dozen plums if I let her.

Charlotte is my trusty helper in the garden with weeding, watering, and harvesting. Because I am color blind, she is an ideal assistant now since she can better identify the ripeness of a fruit. This advantage is counterbalanced by her inability to put berries in any container other than her mouth.

This growing season continues to mete out surprises. Last week the goldenrod (*Solidago*) was blooming; this week the blackberries (*Rubus fruticosus*) start to arrive in the middle of highbush blueberry (*Vaccinium corymbosum*) season. Not that Charlotte is complaining.

Like a ravenous bird, she singularly circles and attacks a berry-laden bush with dexterity and skill, quickly locating the ripest of berries and devouring each one. Though she is right-handed, when picking fruits she displays an ambidextrous skill akin to a berry-picking android.

"Charlotte, where do those berries belong?" I ask.

"They belong in my tummy!" she says holding an empty dish.

"No, they belong in my tummy," I retort.

"No my tummy!"

"No my tummy!"

This repartee can go on forever with Charlotte giggling throughout. But even though our take-home harvest is less than hoped, it pleases me that Charlotte experiences such simple and elemental joy by eating fruit. She prefers fruit to many sweets, though I would not want to force her to choose between a bowl of blueberries and a plate of chocolate-chip cookies.

I appreciate and savor these days with Charlotte. Between snacking in my garden and around our berry bushes, she is eating well and healthy. And like the birds, there will come a season when she doesn't visit us that much anymore, which will increase my harvest and melancholy, because my favorite tiny predator is grown up and has other gardens to explore.

AUGUST OUTING: CLOUD WATCHING

During the languid, slowing days of Summer, sometimes the best activity is no activity. Between the heat and humidity, it is prudent to be economical with movement, particularly in the afternoon. That is why perhaps the backyard is the best place to visit to throw down a blanket and watch the clouds roll by.

High in the sky, fluffy clouds filled with moisture pass by each other, offering their own Rorschach test on imaginations. I see a dragon, you see a claw. You see a candle, I see a sword. Lying on my back, I watch the birds flying overhead, smell the humidity come off the lawn, and start to become sleepy.

HARVESTING BASIL

As Summer's end nears, we wait for the optimal time to harvest. When it comes to basil (*Ocimum basilicum*), I never get the timing right, as this herb often starts sprouting flowers way before I am ready to pick. I don't mind as I find it relaxing pinching off blooms and watching the insects pollinate those I miss. I always plant too much basil as I have great dreams of pesto, and ironically by the end of Summer, I never get around to making enough.

At the Children's Garden we leave much of the harvesting decisions to the students, but sometimes we need to get crops out of the ground quickly for Green Chimneys' clients or just because we need to move on to another piece of the curriculum (and plantings). Last week Tracy and her assistant, Alice, and I spent the better part of the morning pulling up basil plants and picking off all the leaves. Some would be used in the school kitchen immediately and some would be dried in our solar dehydrator for later use.

Standing over the table removing basil leaves, we are quiet, concentrating on the task. The pungent smell of the basil wafts up from our fingers, creating a fragrant space around us. Students join us later in the morning, and one of them starts speaking spontaneously to verbalize her feelings and ideas; soon the rest of the group joins in the discussion. After we harvest all the basil, which is over five pounds, we go our separate ways.

The next day, I realize it is time to harvest the basil in my garden. I consider drying some but my wife cautions me against it as she has always had bad luck doing so. "It always gets moldy. You have to be careful."

I consider this but then remember the solar dehydrator I had just used at the Children's Garden. I come up with a plan. First, I harvest the basil, layering the leaves into cookie trays covered with paper towels. Once the trays are full I place them on a table outside. Around them I place two-by-fours that are slightly higher than the trays. On top of the wood I place old storm windows that complete my make-shift solar oven. I leave and let the sun do its work.

Within an hour the basil has desiccated to half its original size and within three hours it is crispy and ready for harvest. I crush a leaf of dried basil between my fingers to see how well it maintains its smell. Not like fresh basil by any means, but better than store-bought.

POLLINATE ME

When many of the children I work with see an insect, particularly a bee or wasp, their reaction ranges between alarm and outright panic. But one child I work with looks at bees with total indifference.

We are planting a row of lettuce (*Lactuca sativa*) today for Fall harvest, and a fat honey bee flies around our heads and falls to the ground. Jim points it out and says, "That bee looks funny. Is it hurt?"

I stop my seeding and examine it. Its legs are laden with pollen but it is rolling around in the dirt, appearing disoriented. If it were a person, I would have said that he was drunk. I tell Jim I don't know why the bee is behaving that way, but we should let it alone and perhaps it will rest and find its way back to the hive. We watch it, and in a few minutes it regains its footing and flies away.

Going home after teaching at Green Chimneys, I think about the bee and all the different pollinators at work in our gardens. Surveying the different flowers around my house, I notice the variety of pollinators out today. August is a time when many plants are in full bloom waiting for a bug or a breath of wind to move pollen from one flower to another, enabling reproduction.

I am struck by the differences in scents and their potency. The strongest scent in my garden today comes from the white oakleaf hydrangea (*Hydrangea quercifolia*) that is adjacent to my driveway. Its heady bouquet hits me from ten feet away; up close it is overwhelming. The driveway is covered with a dusty white film that has been either discharged or dislodged from its florets. The hydrangea is filled with different insects, each trying to claim as much turf as possible.

The activity around the butterfly bushes (*Buddleia davidii*) is not nearly as frenetic, with bees spending more time around the flowers than butterflies. The purple flowers are headier than the blue ones; the yellows have only a slight scent that is difficult to detect. Not surprisingly, the yellows are the wallflowers of the pollination dance with only a few stragglers looking to take them for a spin.

There is lots of competition for attention in the garden. Our rose of Sharon (*Hibiscus syriacus*) seems to have the worst luck, as its flowers have little scent and few pollinators. The flower of a hosta (*Hosta*) requires the bees and other potential pollinators to wiggle into it as would a youthful camper a sleeping bag. Appearing chaste, hostas hide their anthers and stigmas more than others in the garden.

Sunflowers (*Helianthus annuus*), on the other hand, exclaim, "Pollinate me!" with yellow petals pointing to a landing pad that becomes sticky yellow with excessive organic matter. Bees fight for a place, leaping over the base and becoming insect versions of enormous cargo planes laden with pollen headed for home. Clematis (*Clematis*) is different, as only a few tiny insects attempt to dine on its dainty reproductive parts. A lone hummingbird quickly samples the fuchsia (*Fuchsia*) and then speeds away as quickly as it came.

One advantage our yard has over those of our neighbors is a deer fence that keeps our flowers intact, making our home an oasis for pollinating creatures. They come to dance, eat, and fly from flower to flower before returning to their hives or nests for the evening.

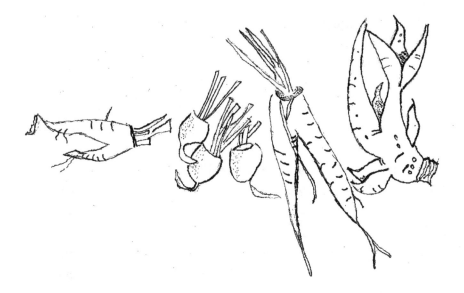

TINY SEEDS, MONSTER CARROTS

My students in the Children's Garden love to harvest the vegetables that they have planted as seeds. They are often astounded when these tiny orbs metamorphose a few months later into food to eat. Observing the transformation between seed and vegetable is especially wondrous to them with carrots, as the seed is minuscule and the resulting root is large.

To start, it takes a great deal of concentration and dexterity to sow carrot seeds properly. But sowing them properly is not necessarily the focus when you work with certain types of children. Some drop a small handful on the ground or toss them into a furrow. Others seek perfection and demand a proxy for measurement so they can understand how much space is needed between seeds. A piece of bark, a twig, a stone. Anything will work.

Within a few weeks, the first hairy green sprigs emerge from the ground, following the patterns of the prior sowing: Sometimes a sparsely planted row appears, other times a thick clump of hairy greens pops up. Once they see the sprigs, the students want to know if the carrots are ready for picking. I tell Selena to grab one and see. She pulls out a tiny root and is disappointed and puzzled. The class erupts with questions.

"Why is it so small?"

"Why isn't it orange?"

"What are these little hairs?"

"When will I get a carrot?"

I tell Selena and the other children that they need to be patient and wait for them to grow, much like they themselves will grow over time and become adults as large as myself. Some are satisfied with that answer, others are indifferent to this reality and want their carrot now.

As the weeks roll on and the tops get larger, it becomes time to thin out the carrots, which requires both care and judgment. The child chosen for this task needs to discriminate between plants and estimate how much space should exist between different carrots as they mature. It can be frustrating for some children, as they expect to pull a carrot they can eat but instead pull a tiny, white, string-like root.

During the next thinning exercise, an identifiable carrot emerges. The thinned carrots can now be eaten, as they resemble the mature ones we will begin to harvest within a month.

In a month, pulling each fully grown carrot from the ground produces a surprise. In anticipation, the children invariably ask questions before each pull.

"How big will it be?

Will I break the top off accidentally?

What will it look like?"

There is no easy way to know by looking at the top. The actual size and shape of the carrot is hidden under the soil. Once the carrots emerge, the students voice their discoveries.

"Whoa, look at the size of this baby!"

"This is so tiny."

"There's nothing here."

Carlos pulls up a carrot that has sprouted what appears to be a pair of legs. And for every twenty carrots we pick, one is misshaped in a weird and unique way.

"These are monster carrots!" says Joan. I ask if they are scary and if she will eat them. She says that she will eat them and they are not scary. I then ask if she ever saw anything like them in a supermarket. She thinks for a moment and then says no, but she wishes stores would sell them as they are "way cool."

Joan then asks me why they vary. I tell her that in certain ways carrots are like people in that each one has the potential to be very different. Some are tall, others are short. Some are thin, others are fat. In our garden the reason for this difference is most likely because the soil contains stones, which interfere with the shape of the carrot as it grows. I also tell Joan that bugs called root-knot nematodes can cause carrots to fork and differ from their ideal inverted conical form.

We harvest the carrots, putting them into two piles: one for the regular boring carrots and another for the special carrots with personality. We wash them after we finish and put them in the refrigerator to be taken later in the day to the kitchen.

THE LIGHTNESS OF BEING CHARD

One of the concepts that is always hard to grapple with, regardless of age, is the idea of weight and volume. A huge tote of lettuce, for example, will likely weigh much less than a small watermelon. When we dig and transport soil, aggregate, stone, or mulch, the children I teach often believe that they can transport much more material in a wheelbarrow than is possible for them.

The best way to teach them how to judge how much something weighs in these cases is to let them lift the wheelbarrow and push it to our destination. Often, particularly with boys, what starts out with great enthusiasm about loading up a wheelbarrow comes crashing down when they have to lift it up. They then need to unload at least half before they can move the wheelbarrow with a modicum of control. And still it takes a few attempts to get them to understand the amount of soil they can handle comfortably.

These ideas come to the fore in the Children's Garden while harvesting Swiss chard (*Beta vulgaris* subsp. *vulgaris*). Swiss chard is one of those great vegetables that keeps on giving. Once it is harvested, it often grows back and delivers at least one more crop. It is one of the few greens that is going gangbusters this year, unbothered by slugs, fungus, or mold. With pruning shears in hand, we go to cull the second crop of chard from the row. It is a good exercise as it requires a child to handle a tool and determine which two leaves not to cut, so the plant can continue to regenerate. We always underestimate the tote needed to hold the harvested chard. At the same time, we decide to pull carrots and bring a different tote for them. We work quietly and quickly in the garden as Rohit has mastered harvesting skills this Summer.

When we finish our harvests, I ask Rohit to guess the weight of the chard and carrots. He picks up the tote and says that the chard weighs at least fifteen pounds and perhaps even twenty. We ask Tracy to eyeball the weight and she says fifteen pounds sounds about right. The carrots, say Rohit, are around five pounds. I think that is a pretty accurate guess, and then we weigh our produce.

Ironically Rohit is almost spot on with the carrots (they weigh six pounds) but we are all way off on the chard (it is only ten pounds). Our problem stems from the fact that our brains confuse volume and weight. Because the chard fills up a twenty-gallon tote, we assume that it must weigh much more than it does. Ah, how the eyes so often deceive.

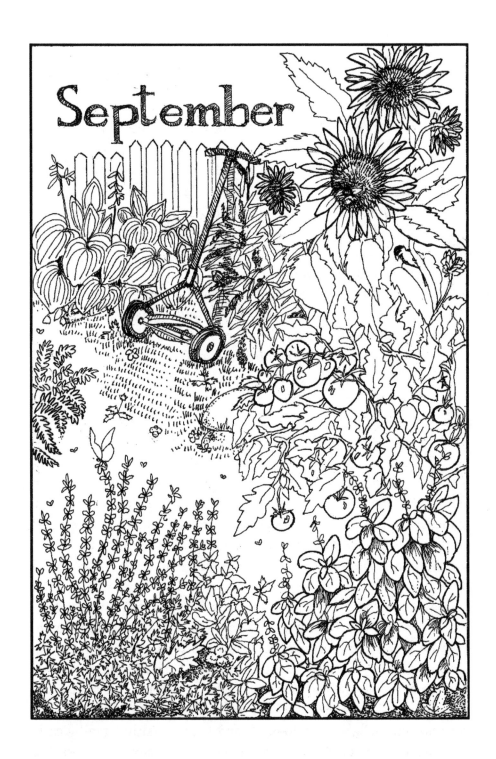

September

SEPTEMBER: HARVEST TIME

September is a bittersweet month as Summer ends and Fall begins. It is the time when the largest bounties of the gardens' flowers, vegetables, and fruits are harvested. Some leaves begin to turn to orange, yellow, and red, while migrating birds and monarch butterflies make their way south.

It is time to bring the outdoor furniture into the shed, garage, or basement. The full harvest moon reminds us that days are shortening and the evening chill in the air will only become more pronounced as the month progresses.

EXTENDING HARVEST TIMES

The counterbalancing forces of the old and new hit hard upon returning to the Children's Garden in September. On the old side, there is the garden, which often enough is in the final throes of harvest and ready to lie fallow. But this year things are a little different. A new program has flipped our perspective and some of our common assumptions.

Earlier this year we started a three-season garden, with a hoped-for Fall harvest into December and an early-Spring harvest in March. We were inspired by pure chance. Last year around this time one of my students found a package of mustard green (*Brassica juncea*) seeds lying around and she wanted to plant them. Neither Tracy nor I saw any harm in the exercise and with her seeded one-half a row. To our surprise and delight, they took off and became fairly large by early November, with colorful red and green leaves ready to harvest. We considered cutting them down for the kitchen, but one project trumped another and by mid December they were blanketed with snow.

By mid March, however, the mustard greens started to reemerge and by April became a row bulging with vegetation ready for the picking. Tracy, I, and the children were amazed by this unlikely survival, as we hadn't done anything to protect them; they had just been left out to fend for themselves against the elements. This success and my rereading of Eliot Coleman's books on four-season harvests led me to suggest to Tracy that we could extend our curriculum to work the garden an additional three months.

Rather than putting the garden to bed, we are waking it up and constructing Agribon hoop houses over the rows to protect our crops that we planted in August. The lettuce (*Lactuca sativa*) we planted in July is ready to be picked; we will trim the leaves so that we can get another crop in a few months. Most of our crops to harvest in November and December are in the soil, sprouting new growth, and I'm looking forward to showing the kids that gardening in the North can be a year-round activity. The kids are bewildered by the idea that we will be growing vegetables through Fall, but I believe they will get into it.

The extended season is just one of the changes going on for me at the garden. I have other unexpected seedlings: new students.

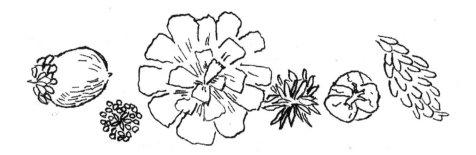

NEW AND OLD SEEDLINGS

The garden in September is time to pick Summer fruits and start a new crop of students. While some of my kids seem to be perennials, over half are new and, like plants in the garden, must be tended with care.

First introductions are always a challenge. I never know the best composition of "soil and light" needed to get a student to bloom. Some children do well with delicate tasks such as sowing carrots, while others excel at moving large piles of soil in wheelbarrows. Regardless, initial impressions are everlasting, and I want to excite and empower the children during our first meetings so that they will want to return to work with me in the garden.

Billy is excited to be in the garden; he is effervescent, talkative, and highly motivated. He wants to please everybody and his energy level is so high that he can't get anything done; he just wants to spend all his time talking about his efforts.

"Aren't I doing a great job, Mr. Keller?"

"Absolutely. Now let's focus on putting the spinach (*Spinacia oleracea*) seeds into the ground."

"If I do a great job, I'll get a big pepper (*Capsicum annuum*), right?"

"We'll see. But we have to do the job before we get anything."

"That's for sure. But I'm working well, aren't I?"

This banter monopolizes our entire session. Anytime another student or teacher comes within earshot, he starts telling them about how good a job he is doing. He is a smart and highly capable child, but he just can't contain his emotions. But I discover that if I leave him alone and isolated from other people, including myself, then he is able to refocus all his energy on the tasks at hand.

For instance, we were seeding collard greens (*Brassica oleracea* var. *viridis*) and I needed to speak with one of the other instructors. I gave him a round rock with a diameter of one inch and told him to plant the seeds one inch (or one rock) apart in the furrows we had etched into the soil. He agreed and I left. I was away for over five minutes but was keeping an eye on him from afar and saw that he painstakingly concentrated on his task without talking or interruption. When I came back, he described his progress and I complimented him, "You did a great job here by yourself. I think that deserves an extra carrot when we finish up." He beamed at me and together we finished up planting the greens with a little less talking than is typical.

Clive is my next new charge. He is very talkative and wants to do a good job, but it takes me a few sessions to determine the types of jobs he is best suited for. His reactions change day to day, and he has large mood swings from sad to mad to indifferent to joyful. I discover that he reacts well to simple, focused chores. Today, we need to seed for a Fall-and-Spring harvest, so I have him work with two different types of seeds: lettuce and spinach. I tell him that he needs to place a seed every half inch. He replies that he doesn't know how far a space that represents, so I find a rock with a half-inch diameter and tell him to place each seed a rock's width apart. Clive nods and starts to plant.

He finds it difficult to hold the seeds with one hand and plant them with the other. I offer to hold the seeds while he plants them. Clive agrees and together we plant a neat row of lettuce. He continues this for quite a few rows. I ask him why he likes to plant seeds and he responds, "It keeps me calm. I'm happy when I do this."

We seed an entire section of a garden bed with me holding the seeds and Clive dropping them into the slight furrows we have made with the end of a rake. I make attempts at conversation, but Clive is better focused in silence. Singing birds and the far-away voices of other children are our only audible stimulation. When finished I say, "Now we need to tuck them into their bed, like you would put a blanket on a baby. So take your hands with palms down and move the soil over the seeds like this," I tell him as I demonstrate the technique. He nods his head and finishes tucking in the seeds quickly, happy that this activity is over.

We now turn to plant the spinach seeds. We work together in the same way but he masters the distance of half an inch and discards the spacing stone. We work deftly, seeding our rows, finishing with time to spare.

Ironically, Clive appears uninterested in harvesting anything from the garden to eat. This surprises me because most children enjoy grabbing snacks from the soil after a job well done. In an attempt to change his mind, I walk him through the garden identifying all the different plants and vegetables that are ready to be picked (and eaten).

He does not react as we walk through the onions (*Allium cepa*) and lettuce. Clive's indifference fades, however, as we walk through the tomatoes (*Solanum lycopersicum*); when he spots a pink princess cherry tomato he suddenly becomes interested in harvesting and pops a couple into his mouth while agreeing to pick more for the kitchen. "This isn't so bad," says Clive as he munches on this small fruit.

My next student is attending a special meeting so I have a free period and return to the garden. When I arrive a group of preschoolers are walking around with their teachers. I ask them if they would like to do something special and they all say yes. I take them to a corner of the herb garden where there is a large patch of woolly thyme (*Thymus pseudolanuginosus*).

"Take both of your hands, palms out like this," I say and show. "And then rub the thyme and smell your fingers." The group stands bent over the thyme, with hands and backsides wiggling, unable to stop their fingers from rubbing the soft, wool-like plant. They soon smell their fingers and start to giggle.

Next to the woolly thyme is our mint (*Mentha*) patch, so I remove a stem and give a leaf to each child and tell them to smell it. "It smells like gum," says a little girl. "Can we eat it?" asks another.

I tell them that they can, and then I break off a small branch and start to tickle each of their noses with it. "Tickle my nose again!" insists a bespectacled girl. We then walk over to a patch of sunflowers (*Helianthus annuus*). One sunflower plant has pollinated flowers and an adjacent one does not, offering me a chance to explain how seeds are created. I cut open each flower showing them the difference between the two. "Each little flower on the big circle needs to be pollinated by a bug to create a seed," I say. "After a bug touches it the right way, the plant makes a seed."

"You see each of these holes?" I say, pointing at the other sunflower. "Each used to hold a seed like it was in a tiny little bed. Each seed can grow into a plant that is this tall." I point to our sunflowers, some of which are ten feet high. The children are amazed that such a tiny seed can grow into such a large plant. "Does anyone want a seed to grow a sunflower next Spring?" I ask. Everyone says yes and I place a seed into each tiny waiting hand.

SEPTEMBER CRAFT: COLLECT NUTS AND CONES FOR WINTER PROJECTS

Making pine-cone wreaths, bird feeders, and other Winter decorations is a fun craft for later in the year. However, the raw materials for these exercises must be collected before they are gathered and eaten by animals or covered by snow.

Acorns can start to fall as early as August, but always before the leaves begin to drop, making September a prime time to collect these nuts from oaks (Quercus). Other nut-bearing trees to watch out for include hickory (Carya), walnut (Juglans), and buckeye (Aesculus glabra). Cones, and not just the pine (Pinus) variety, are also available this time of year. If you wait too long, it is difficult to find undamaged samples. Taking a walk in the woods with a few paper bags for collection is a quiet and reflective way to appreciate the waning warmth.

THE EXISTENTIAL PLEASURES OF THE UNFAMILIAR

One of the things I find most gratifying when working at the Children's Garden is introducing students to familiar friends of mine that they have never seen or experienced. This was the case when we replaced our loud, noisy, and dangerous gas mower with a Scotts sixteen-inch reel model.

A manual mower doesn't spout fumes or much noise but emits a quiet whirl of the blades scraping the cutting bar as it severs the grass.

It is so quiet that I can mow my lawn in the early morning without disturbing anyone in the neighborhood.

I see little frogs, toads, and other creatures that hop out of the way as I mow the lawn. I have enough control over my machine that I don't frappe them. I can also hear what is happening around me as I make the circular hike about my yard. I thought that this would be a good addition to the Children's Garden and that the students would take to it.

Tracy is dubious at first when I suggest the switch. I predict that the children will gladly take over our mowing chore as they will be fascinated by such an atypical tool. Once we receive the mower, Tracy discovers how correct I am.

"My god. That's all they want to do," laughs Tracy after the mower is assembled and put to use. "The lawn gets mowed two or three times a day now." It doesn't really matter that the kids don't mow in a straight line or follow a regimented pattern. When you mow an area a few times a day, everything will be cut eventually.

I was able to extend this lesson to one of my students. Paul is a unique child in that he hunts deer with his father and knows how to drive his uncle's John Deere tractor; he also mows lawns, shovels snow, and rakes leaves for extra money. Reminds me of the jobs I had as a young man.

"Have you ever used a mower like this before?" I ask.

"Nope," he replies. "This looks pretty old-fashioned."

"Well, yeah, but do you think you are strong enough to handle it?"

He gives me a knowing smile and then grabs its handle. Paul gives it an initial push and seems a little shocked at the ease with which it travels the ground, sending up a tiny wave of grass clippings that land by his feet. He walks to the end of a vegetable row accompanied by the gentle sound of the blades severing the grass and then turns around to return. He has a big smile on his face. "This takes some work, but it's a lot of fun."

"If you want to do a really good job, you need to watch your line and overlap where the blades cut the grass so you don't miss any parts." I show him how to navigate a turn to overlap a line of uncut grass. He nods, takes over and starts to concentrate. His eye is trained on the wheel and the line of uncut grass as he walks up and down the lawn area in the garden. He looks determined as he guides the mower carefully so that he does not waste any amount of his cut.

Paul soon falls into a groove. A restful, happy look beams from his face. I sit on an old bucket watching him mow the lawn with the only sound in the background being a few twittering birds and the rhythmic swish of the mower reel slicing off the blades of remaining grass.

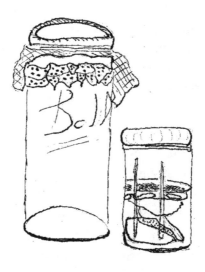

SECOND TIME SWEET

This is the second consecutive year that I have run a class on flavored vinegars at Ann's Place. Last year's activity attracted a large crowd who loved all the different flavors we were able to concoct. But I need to add a twist to keep it interesting for repeat clients. I hope the addition of an artisanal vinegar "mother" will pique their interest.

As the class enters the kitchen area, I place the mother, a gelatinous, cream-colored blob of bacteria that is used to create vinegar, in the middle of the table surrounded by a sampling of vinegars.

"While many of you may think that vinegar is a simple item, there are many different options and possibilities in its creation," I start. "We'll be making flavored vinegars later, but I'd like to challenge your tastes by having you sample a group of artisanal vinegars made by a monk at a local monastery. I will also let you contrast these vinegars against a flavored one I made last year."

With that I lay out fresh bread that I had baked that morning and the vinegars: red wine, apple cider, sherry, apricot, white wine and raspberry artisan vinegars, and my homemade flavored vinegar. I pour a small sample of each into a glass bowl, leaving the bottle adjacent.

I advise my clients, "First smell the contents of the bottle to see if you can discern the different flavors by smell, then try a few drops on a piece of bread or in a spoon." Different facial expressions emerge from my clients' faces as they discern the subtle characteristics of each vinegar.

"I can really taste the apricot."

"The sherry is too strong for me."

"Is this apple cider? It's wonderful."

Ironically, my clients point to the vinegar that I made over a year ago as their favorite. Many prefer it over the vinegars made with the mother by the brother at the monastery. The recipe I used for my vinegar is a combination of parsley (*Petroselinum crispum*), sage (*Salvia officinalis*), rosemary (*Salvia rosmarinus*), and thyme (*Thymus vulgaris*) that are infused in common white vinegar. It's what I call the Simon & Garfunkel recipe.

"Now that you've tasted the different types of vinegars, let's go outside to the herb garden and choose the herbs to flavor yours," I say. "I've also brought champagne grapes (*Vitis vinifera*) and fresh cloves (*Syzygium aromaticum*) as well as blackberries (*Rubus fruticosus*), and blueberries (*Vaccinium corymbosum*) from my garden."

The addition of raised-bed herb gardens at Ann's Place has dramatically increased the therapeutic options for my clients. They often walk among the mints (*Mentha*) and other herbs, scratching and sniffing for relief and solace. As clients start to stuff their jars with different herbs to infuse, I notice that one person is choosing St. John's wort (*Hypericum perforatum*) from the medicinal-herb raised bed, which also has sage, chamomile (*Matricaria chamomilla*), horehound (*Marrubium vulgare*), and comfrey (*Symphytum officinale*).

"That may not be a good thing to include in your infusion as it is used to treat depression, insomnia, and anxiety. Perhaps chamomile is a better choice," I suggest.

She nods and looks toward other plants.

After the group finishes collecting their herbs, we return to the kitchen. Fragrant, fresh German red garlic (*Allium senescens*) from my garden is a popular addition to many concoctions. Bugs and detritus are carefully removed from the herbs before we pour near-boiling white vinegar into each mason jar holding their collections. Vapors from the vinegar burn my eyes slightly before I top off each jar with a canning lid and ring, sealing it with a good twist.

The pouring of vinegar into mason jars reminds me of when my wife and I used to can tomato sauce, peaches, and strawberry jam. But unlike those canning activities, no sweet smell is coming from the pot, tempting me to take a lick, but rather a very sour one. Now that the jars have been filled, it is time to decorate bottles that will be used later to store the vinegar when the infusions are mature.

While my clients last year were more ascetic in their bottle decorations, opting for simple labels and a bow or two, this year they embrace bling. Every little decorative tchotchke that I had purchased as a lark is used. Some of the jars are so covered with decorations, there will be little space left to see the vinegar's final color.

"You should let your vinegar infuse for one to two months," I say. "Take a taste every week or two to see the change in potency. When it's to your liking, strain it a couple of times using a coffee filter and use a plastic or stainless steel funnel to put it into your decorated bottles."

They nod in acknowledgment and continue to cover their bottles with the unclaimed scraps of decorations that litter the counter.

GETTING AND GIVING BACK

Today we harvest vegetables in the Children's Garden that we will deliver to a local food pantry. We first collect all the tomatoes that are on the vines, regardless of ripeness. We only have four plants but are able to glean twenty-five pounds of fruit. We then pull a dozen basil

(*Ocimum basilicum*) plants and place them in a bucket filled with water. The leaves will be removed later. When one child wonders why we are harvesting these plants, I rub a leaf on her nose. At first she is taken aback, but quickly smiles and embraces the scent.

We next gather the Swiss chard (*Beta vulgaris* subsp. *vulgaris*) and leeks (*Allium porrum*) that were pulled yesterday and stored in our refrigerator. Tracy gives me some extra garlic (*Allium sativum*), adds some parsley, and throws in a couple of squashes (*Cucurbita*). We now have over sixty pounds of food to deliver. The students and I get into a small school bus with our vegetables and leave campus.

We have a short and uneventful ride to the pantry, a run-down red brick building on Main Street in Brewster, New York, but once we arrive, the children's excitement can no longer be contained. "I want to hand out all the vegetables we harvested," says Jose.

The pantry's coordinator, Mary, greets us and organizes our group into separating and packing everything we brought in. "Everything needs to be put in a bag," she says. "Why don't we start with the tomatoes?" All the children grab five or six tomatoes to place in plastic bags that will be tied with a wire and placed on the table. We do the same with the Swiss chard and parsley. The garlic is already in tiny braids.

"We get all the food here from supermarkets like Trader Joe's as well as from the government for distribution," says Mary. "But we don't have much fresh food. This is a real treat." The children marvel at not only how tightly everything is packed and organized in a storage area but also by the variety of food and goods available to those in need. Two of the refrigerators on site are stuffed with donated sheet cakes and pies. Non-food items, such as boxes of disposable diapers, rest nearby.

We are hoping that today's recipients will enjoy our selection of straight-from-the-garden produce as a change from their usual fare. Most of the fresh food donated to the pantry is produce that is past its prime. Pears with spots or apples with bruises are okay to donate, but moldy grapes are not. Regardless of condition, however, fresh vegetables and fruits are just a fraction of the shopping bag of staples that the pantry's clients receive as a supplement to their meals. Mary thanks us for the produce we have contributed and for the time we have spent preparing the food for distribution. The children enjoy being instructed how to put together bags of food for the people who come to the center. They feel helpful.

On the way back to school, I ask the children what they have learned today. Bella says, "It was good to help people with our garden." Jose says, "It was great to help so many poor people in such a poor area." I respond, "Why do you think they're poor?"

It is easy to see how he comes to this assumption. The cramped offices are simply appointed with worn and old furniture. Some of the clients picking up bags of food are wearing ripped, old jeans and T-shirts. Elderly patrons thank us for the food we hand to them with grins missing more than a few teeth.

"It's not just poor people who need places like this. Many people today are down on their luck, without jobs, and needing a little help," I say. "We're lucky at our school to have plenty of food and people who take care of you." The children nod. Bella adds, "It's good to give people food so they won't be hungry."

SEPTEMBER OUTING: VISIT A FARM

With harvests in high gear, September is one of the best times to visit a farm. The fields are lush with growth, vegetables, and fruit. It is the cusp of the seasons, between the final gathering of warm-weather crops like corn (Zea mays) and the harvest of potatoes (Solanum tuberosum) and squash in Fall.

Pick-your-own farms let you choose the best tomatoes, peppers, peaches (Prunus persica), and other crops to enjoy immediately or preserve for the months ahead. Canning vegetables and fruits now can help anyone appreciate this delightful month in the dead of Winter when the days are short and the only things growing outside are the shadows and icicles.

AUTUMNAL PLUMS

The harvest and display of flowers is abundant, while their remaining time with us is slight. My mother's rose (*Rosa*) bush is starting its second flowering and the buds on her Montauk daisies (*Nipponanthemum nipponicum*) have blossomed. After I finish the chore I had promised to do for her, I suggest that we take a drive to the beach on this perfect early Fall day. She agrees with a smile.

We drive to Short Beach in Smithtown, New York, where my father used to walk with her a few times every week regardless of the weather or season. We sit on a bench, gazing at Long Island Sound and the Connecticut shoreline, remembering the days when I was a young boy and we came to the beach as a newly transplanted family from Pittsburgh, Pennsylvania. My mother would fill a thermos with hot dogs and boiling water for a beach-side dinner that would be consumed as my younger brother, sister, and I scampered along the beach, looking for horseshoe-crab molts, shells, and pieces of wood we would fashion into a boat to be launched into the Sound.

After a childhood of collecting such detritus on the beach, I have moved on to scavenge other things from the shore. This time of year it is beach plums (*Prunus maritima*). In mid to late September beach-plum season is in full swing on Long Island, so I time my visits to my mother to take full advantage of the bounty. Last year the harvest was poor, no doubt due to the cool, rainy, Summer we'd had. When I viewed them in mid August this year, bundles of tiny fruit hung from the branches, promising a future sweet harvest. But in the last month, excessive heat and the lack of rain could well have dashed my hopes; perhaps at the very least there will be a sampling of fruit on the bushes.

As feared, the bushes are distressed, as it has rained less than an inch since I last saw them. Raisin-like bunches of plums hang on branches devoid of leaves. Mostly pit, these little blue orbs are sad decorations portending the beginning of Fall and perhaps the death of the plant.

I do, however, find a few bushes that for some reason are flush with green leaves and fat blue plums. I greedily harvest a bowl of them for my wife and I to consume over the next week.

Beach plums are an acquired taste. They are the size of a gooseberry (*Ribes uva-crispa*), taste like a plum mixed with a wild blueberry (*Vaccinium angustifolium*), and have a large pit similar to that of a cherry (*Prunus avium*). One year my wife Juana and I made beach-plum jam, which was delicious to eat but time consuming to make because of the pitting process. In bountiful years they are our fruit of choice when we feel like a light snack. As you expel pit after pit from your mouth, however, you often wonder if it is worth the effort, as the pit sometimes appears bigger than the fruit you are able to ingest.

The berries have a short table life because they ripen quickly once picked. Some of the plums are still too sour and my color blindness doesn't let me differentiate a sweet ripe plum from a sour unripe one. Others are past their prime and when you bite into them they provide a squirt of fermented juice. These are the most interesting to taste; the little jolts of alcohol remind me of the homemade wine that my father used to receive from a friend.

Sitting on a bench at the beach, I hand a few to my mother as she sits and looks out toward the Sound. She bites into a plum and makes a sour face. After spitting out the pit she says, "Your father would have liked this." We sit for a while without words, watching the seagulls fly overhead, inhaling the salty breeze coming off the water in the late afternoon.

DRYING TIME

Late September is when the herb garden and mint walk get harvested at Ann's Place. The first sub-forty-degree temperatures have not hit yet, and all the leaves are still fresh for use, but their days are numbered. Few clients dry their own herbs so this is a good opportunity to expand their horizons. I pass out a half dozen paper bags to each client, many of whom have brought a pruner as I suggested.

"Now is not the best time to be harvesting herbs," I tell them as we walk out to the gardens midafternoon. "The best time is early morning after the dew has dried and it has not become too hot. But the herbs should be okay to harvest as it rained last night and it's cloudy today. There should be lots of moisture in all the leaves.

"On your right is the mint walk. On your left are our herbal gardens. Everything is labeled. Before you start choosing which herbs to select, take some time to smell them and consider what you want to use them for."

My clients comply and start to scratch and sniff all the different herbs and mints.

"These mints smell really different." Yes, we have over fifteen varieties.

"Are you sure about this thyme? It smells like oregano (*Origanum vulgare*)." Yes, it's oregano thyme, a special variety.

"Can I use St. John's wort and comfrey for tea?" Yes, but use them sparingly and know what you want to use them for, because they treat different ailments.

Roberta has come to the class looking a little sad and preoccupied, but after a few minutes over the herb beds her spirits are lifted, evidenced by a big smile on her face.

"There are lots of different ways to dry herbs and mints," I say. "Perhaps the easiest way is to cut long stems off the plants and hang them upside down in a paper bag. That way all the oils run into the leaves and the leaves are protected from the sun. You can bundle the ends with string or a rubber band. Pop a few air holes in the paper bag for ventilation and you are done."

I give everyone an instruction sheet as well as other tips and techniques for how to dry herbs. Everyone quickly fills the bags I gave them, but I brought extras. One client brought her young son to the class. He looks out of sorts, so I ask him if he would like something to eat. He shyly nods his head and I take his hand, leading him over to our patch of sorrel (*Rumex acetosa*), a favorite of most children. He is indifferent as he starts to nibble on a leaf and then sticks the rest into his mouth, which soon extends into a big grin covered with bits of leaf and spittle. His mother and the rest of the class don't need such encouragement as they scratch, sniff, and collect their way through their garden walk.

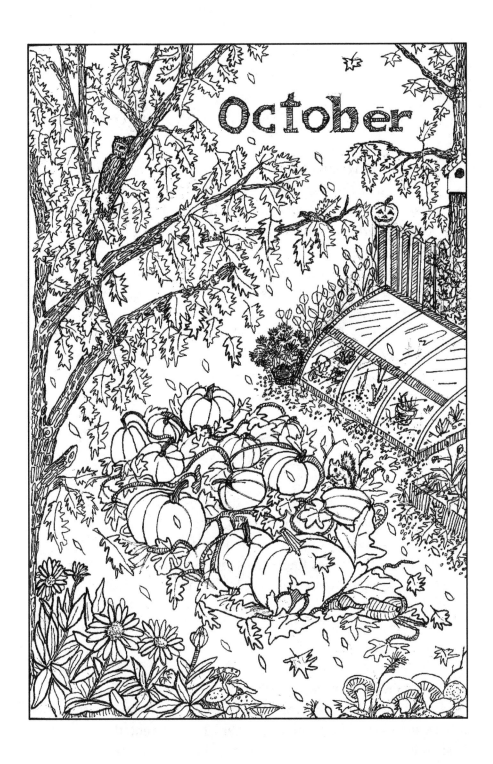

OCTOBER: WINDING DOWN

October's cooling temperatures and fading vegetation represent the last breath of Mother Nature's colorful splendor before dormancy takes over. The sun is accelerating its drop in the sky, casting long and lasting shadows.

Animals ready themselves for the cold months ahead by collecting nuts and other foods frantically. Gardeners and farmers, too, pick up the pace of harvesting, looking to beat frosts or freak snow storms that can hit at the end of the month. Those without such pressing chores have the luxury to enjoy the new colors and pungent scents of the season.

BLIND (COLOR) GARDENING

Picking the remaining tomatoes off the vines with my students at the Children's Garden at Green Chimneys, I have them select twelve red tomatoes (*Solanum lycopersicum*) and line them up by hue. They have lots of fun arguing among themselves the relative positions of the fruits but eventually agree upon their places, light to dark red. Once they are done, I am at a purposeful disadvantage.

"Are these really different colors? They all look the same to me."

My kids are flabbergasted.

"Mr. Keller, don't you see?"

"I can't believe you can't see!"

It is a rare and special moment when you truly connect with a child in a learning situation. Though each person is different, the connection is singular, as each one focuses on you intently, hanging onto each word and expression. It is a wonderful feeling that transcends the typical relationship between student and teacher or mentor. And it can happen anywhere, anytime. A favorite bug is discovered. Bees congregate around a sunflower (*Helianthus annuus*) as huge as a serving plate. A hummingbird flutters by, taking in the nectar of a fuchsia (*Fuchsia*). And a connection always occurs when I let slip my hidden disability: I am color blind.

Color blindness is not unique as an estimated eight percent of males but less than one percent of all females have it. My particular type of color blindness, which affects only one percent of all men, makes it difficult for me to distinguish colors in the green-yellow-red portion of the visible light spectrum; I also see little difference between violet, blue, lavender, and purple. I also have a hard time, depending upon the light, seeing differences between red and brown or gray and pink. I am color-challenged.

The discovery that I am color blind intrigues my students. A barrage of questions ensues.

"What is the color of this?" they say repeatedly, pointing to different objects.

"Can you see color?"

"Is all you see black and white?"

After we get through the initial set of queries, my students and I return our focus to the task at hand. This new knowledge, however, changes their view toward the lesson. Now they are very engaged, as my inability to distinguish the tomatoes' color has put them in the driver's seat for this session.

Even though students often take the lead working in the Children's Garden, the fact that I am unable to offer any opinion on the color of the tomatoes they are selecting and how they are being organized is empowering. They become the teacher and I follow their lead.

Sorting through fruits, some students desire a more detailed explanation of how I became color blind and how the world appears to me. "Color blindness is hereditary. In my case, it was passed from my mother to me. She got it from her father, my grandfather, who was color blind," I say. "I've been told that he was so color blind that he used only blue bulbs to decorate the Christmas tree and the exterior of his house." As for the second part of the question, the best explanation I have come up with is to ask my students if they have ever been to a paint store and seen the rack holding all the paper paint swatches. Nearly all nod their heads yes.

"Well to me, instead of seeing thousands of different colors, with each paper representing a different shade, I just see many papers all the same color. Even though the reds and browns, for example, typically are placed far apart in different sections, to me they all look the same.

"As to how the world looks to me, I can't describe it to you, but I think it's probably much less colorful. You can see shades of color that I can never imagine. That's why you should always look closely to see all the different things you can in the garden." With that they are satisfied, and for most of our session together they become very protective of me.

I have been told when working with special-needs children that you should guard your privacy carefully and not let them know much about your personal life. But revealing my visual disability to my students strengthened our connection and showed them that I am as human as they are, with problems that can be overcome with a little bit of help and kindness.

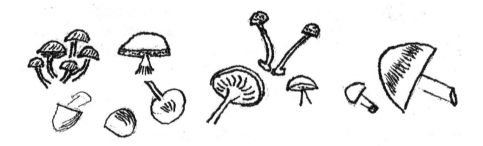

MY LOVE-HATE RELATIONSHIP
WITH GARLIC MUSTARD

Decades ago when I was an occasional rather than an obsessive gardener, I discovered this tiny plant in the backyard that would send up the most delicate little white flower in Spring and then large heart-

and kidney-shaped leaves in Summer. To me it was beautiful, creating waves of leaves that undulated over a densely shaded hill. At the time it seemed a good idea to let it flourish, as it would cover otherwise barren areas of our garden with a blanket of toothy, deep green leaves.

I am reminded of that time this Fall. My clients and I at Ann's Place continue to pull that plant from the garden before it dies off and becomes dormant, only to reemerge in Spring to flower and reproduce. For years I let it flower and spread with abandon in my yard and surrounding woods, not knowing that one of our more invasive plants, garlic mustard (*Alliaria petiolata*), was slowly taking over large portions of our lot, choking off native flowers and plants. By the time I figured it out, it had smothered everything else I was trying to grow in certain areas.

Now, I could have decided to cultivate this biennial imported from Europe in the nineteenth century, because its seeds, stalks, leaves, and roots are edible. There are recipes for pesto and garlic mustard in lemon sauce. It also has medicinal uses. But my family nixed this idea. They are tired of me experimenting on their stomachs with "weird vegetables," though I am able to slip in tiny leaves of garlic mustard for early Spring wild salads. My clients are of a similar ilk, as most of them find the leaves too bitter for their palate.

When I am in the garden with clients, the question, "What is a weed?" often comes up, and the answer is always, "A weed is a plant that you don't want in a given space." If you have a tomato plant in a spinach (*Spinacia oleracea*) patch, it is a weed.

For me, garlic mustard, unlike poison ivy (*Toxicodendron radicans*), can't be categorized easily. Clearing a section at Ann's Place, I leave a few for a snack next year.

PRUNING EXPECTATIONS

Introducing new tools to special-needs children can be challenging. You never know how much experience or aptitude they have, and you are always apprehensive as to how well and, more importantly, how safely they can use what you place in their hands. Even something as elemental as a shovel may be new to them. In certain circumstances it can be turned into a weapon. Such concerns come to mind today in the Children's Garden as stevia (*Stevia rebaudiana*) and sage (*Salvia officinalis*) are being cut to dry. Some lettuce (*Lactuca sativa*) also needs to be harvested.

Cutting stevia and sage to dry is straightforward: Remove two-thirds of the growth off each plant, collect a small bundle of branches, tie the branches together, and then hang them in the shed to dry. Alec has no trouble with the chore or the tool. After I show him the locking mechanism of the Felco #6 (a smaller version of the #2) pruners I give him, he is able to determine where to cut, how to organize the cuttings, and how to bundle them after being trimmed. He is a natural at it, and even though it is the first time he has used pruners, he masters the tool quickly.

But William is entirely different. The locking mechanism of the pruners perplexes him. Initially he can't figure out how to open the pruner by engaging the locking mechanism. I need to demonstrate the action of the pruner and assist William quite a few times before he can open and close it with ease. Then it is time to cut, but William has difficulty understanding what it means to prune two-thirds of the length of a branch.

I change the cut length to one-half of the branch but to no avail. William still is unable to complete this task, necessitating more direct involvement on my part.

I move next to William and hold a branch, telling him to cut it below where my fingers are holding the plants. In the beginning, this is a little risky as William finds it difficult to steady the cutting blades of the pruners. Sometimes he is six inches off, other times the blades come dangerously close to my fingers. But after about twenty cuts, he is able to cut the branches safely about an inch below my fingers. I take the sage branches and drop them into a small pile adjacent to us.

When we have cut enough sage, I tell William to take four branches, match the ends together and then hold the bunch so I can tie it up. He looks at me, says, "Fine," and then tosses the pruner aside.

"William, why did you toss the pruner?" Nothing. He stares outward blankly. I pick up the pruner.

"Please, William, look at the pruner. What do you see?"

At first he says nothing, looking downward. He then mutters, "Dirt and stuff."

"That's right, and that dirt and stuff will clog the pruner and make the blades dull. Remember what I told you before? When you finish using the pruner, you lock the blade and then put it in your pocket."

He nods. I have him clean the blades with a paper towel, lock the pruner, and place it into his pocket. We then tie bundles of sage. He walks back to his class subdued.

Then there is George. Like Alec, George figures out the mechanics of the pruner quickly and uses it to harvest some lettuce. But when we stop to take a break, George takes out the pruner and places the skin between his thumb and index finger between the blades of the pruner.

"George," I say in a firm but calm manner. "What you are doing now isn't safe. Stop." He follows my instruction, but within a minute he repeats his prior action. I remove the pruner before he hurts himself.

"Okay, George. Why don't we mix it up? I'll cut the lettuce and you place it in the bin." He agrees that this is a good idea; it helps that the lettuce we need to harvest is in the center of the row and hard for him to reach without stepping in the garden. We finish our activity without incident, but I inform Tracy that George should be watched carefully when given a tool and that for the time being he should not be given pruners.

OCTOBER CRAFT: COLLECT SEEDS

In early October as the number of fading flowers increase, so do the number of seeds that are ready for harvesting. Those from plants we admire can be collected in a pre-dormancy state, ready to spring to life with water, soil, and patience.

Oak trees (Quercus) have fat acorns while astilbes (Astilbe) and lupines (Lupinus) have tiny, imperceptible seeds. The last lingering fruits can be collected and dried to reveal seeds to be sowed in Spring. Wax paper sandwich bags or seed packets can store and separate these collections for seasons to come.

INDIAN FALL

Juana, Charlotte, and I walk into town to visit the local farmer's market. The day's unusual warmth is counterbalanced by falling leaves and seasonal colors. There are only a few stands with produce, but they are thoroughly stocked. We are expecting Fall crops of peppers (*Capsicum annuum*), potatoes (*Solanum tuberosum*), kale (*Brassica oleracea* var. *sabellica*), and Brussels sprouts (*Brassica oleracea* var. *gemmifera*). But added to these are tomatoes, corn (*Zea mays*), raspberries (*Rubus idaeus*), and other crops more indicative of late August than mid October.

Perhaps their availability is due to an unusual stretch of weather in which a cool, wet August combined with a warm, dry September and October. In the early 1990s we used to get hard frosts at our Connecticut home in late September–early October. This year it appears that we won't get a frost until November. The warmth reminds me of Long Island. Even though it is just a little more than forty miles south of us, it is a good ten to fifteen degrees warmer due to its proximity to the water and our current home's altitude of 840 feet above sea level on a north-facing hill.

By this time of year we used to have Indian Summer days, a warm spell after the first killing frost. We haven't gotten close with only a few early mornings dropping to the high thirties. This weather is in contrast to that described by *New York Times* journalist Hal Borland, who penned columns from the 1940s through the 1970s describing Nature and the changing seasons of northwest Connecticut. In his time, late September and early October columns are about Jack Frost painting the landscape; he couldn't write those observations today.

It is with mixed emotions that I embrace this weather. The wood is too difficult to split as it has yet to freeze solid. Female mosquitoes continue to swarm outside looking for, perhaps, their last drink of blood. The days are warm enough to continue to wear shorts and bicycle on trails that are becoming harder to discern because of the leaf cover. My wool vest is too warm to wear outside, and most evenings are too warm for a fire in the stove.

THE UNCOMMON GREENS OF FALL

My family has been gently indulgent of my attempt to expand the fresh vegetable and salad season into late Fall and Winter. Their comments to me are soothing albeit insincere affirmations.

"I'm sure everything will come out great, Erik."

"Oh, that's nice Dad."

"I'm looking forward to it."

I realize that I am fighting against common wisdom rather than malice. No one wishes me ill, but rather they believe my desire to provide a consistent supply of greens throughout the year is a Quixotic quest. As I have been unable to convince any of them to become my trusty Sancho-like companion, I have to pursue this "impossible dream" on my own.

Candidly, they do have reasons to be skeptical.

Last year I constructed a greenhouse and doubled my space of raised beds, promising food aplenty.

It was a bust.

But as there are no failures in the garden, I realized why I was without greens last Fall and how I could remedy the issue this year. Determined not to be accused again of tilting at horticultural windmills, my first change was not to seed directly into the beds. What I discovered last year was that when you have large slugs in the garden, which you do in September, seedlings have no chance at all to get beyond the early germination stages.

Carefully planted lettuce and spinach seeds would pop up in the garden, forming nice rows, only to be wiped out in a single evening by slugs, slimy versions of Jabba the Hut in both corpulence and appetite.

By the time I discovered the pests, the season and potential for greens were over.

This year I started all my greens in the greenhouse in August, contained in flats. Before I transferred them to the garden, they grew large enough to stand a chance against the slugs and other pests. I also put down iron phosphate, an organic poison for slugs.

And it has worked. I have a cold frame full of plants in different sizes and growths that should permit us to harvest greens throughout Fall and perhaps again in Spring. I ask my wife if she wants a fresh salad for lunch. Juana says that would be nice, but we don't have any greens in the fridge.

"I'll get some from the garden." I harvest some sorrel (*Rumex acetosa*), parsley (*Petroselinum crispum*), thyme (*Thymus vulgaris*), nasturtium (*Tropaeolum majus*) flowers, arugula (*Eruca vesicaria* subsp. *sativa*), romaine (*Lactuca sativa* var. *longifolia*), mizuna (*Brassica juncea* var. *japonica*), corn salad (*Valerianella locusta*) and mesclun, a seed mix of various greens. I wash them, add some goat cheese, and serve the salad to my wife. Juana is in love.

"This is so fresh! It's incredible!"

Later I make a dinner salad for the entire family. They think it wonderfully fresh, and when I tell them that it comes from the garden, they are pleasantly surprised. Hopefully they realize that I have slain a giant and have not been tilting at windmills.

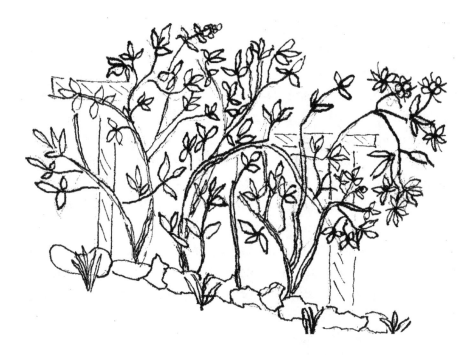

THE EXISTENTIAL PLEASURES OF BUILDING TRELLISES

Over the past two weeks my students have been united in their interest and enthusiasm to build a series of trellises for raspberries and blackberries (*Rubus fruticosus*).

In the Children's Garden, one plot of ground is sloped and not hospitable to plants. Last year's introduction of highbush blueberry bushes (*Vaccinium corymbosum*) is a failure; the soil has a high clay content and was not acidic enough. On the other hand, the cuttings of gooseberry bush (*Ribes uva-crispa*) I planted last year took well and should fruit this coming Spring. Gooseberries are a favorite fruit of the children.

We decide that we should give raspberries and blackberries a chance in this area as they tend to grow well in any type of soil. To maximize our space, Tracy comes up with a rough design of the type of trellis she wants; it is up to me and my students to create a parts list as well as construct the trellises.

The first part of the project is to determine what we need. Tom and I sit down with Tracy's drawing of the proposed trellis and decide to make it six feet high and three feet wide in the shape of a T. We also measure how far apart we will place the different posts used to support the wires that the berry vines will rest upon. I turn the measurements into a mathematics lesson. One child can multiply but cannot add; other children have the opposite problem.

The following week Tracy gets us the lumber and concrete mix we need; it's now time to dig holes. The ground in our garden is filled with compacted loam and clay. A traditional post-hole digger will be difficult for the kids to use, so I bring my father's post-hole auger to grind out the dirt. When we start the job, every child wants to use the auger. It looks like a giant drill bit with a big handle on top to turn; they have never seen anything like it before. Once they use it they are amazed how well it can dig a perfectly round hole. And every child asks the same set of questions:

"How far down do we need to go Mr. Keller?"

"To the line marked on the handle," I reply, pointing to a taped mark I made twenty-seven inches from the tip of the auger.

"That's too much. I'll never be able to do it."

I assure each child that we will work together to dig the hole and together we will accomplish our task. When they get tired, I take over, but within a minute or two of rest each child is ready to resume work. The novelty of the auger trumps fatigue, real or perceived. Each has a different technique. Some lean into the auger hard and turn it slowly. Others opt to spin it quickly. And others spin around with the auger, making me dizzy just watching them work. Regardless of technique or child, it takes about twenty to thirty minutes to dig a hole.

One girl, Sharron, doesn't believe she is strong enough to use the auger. She looks sad and upset that she will not be able to participate.

"Sharron, why don't you and Emily work together, each on different sides of the handle?" I suggest. Emily is a good friend that Sharron likes to be paired with. Both children smile, and after some instruction they walk in a tight circle following each other. They giggle and go faster and faster without getting dizzy. In no time, their hole is dug, ready for the post to be set in concrete.

Most of the children take the challenge of setting the posts very seriously, working diligently to keep each one stable and straight using a level while I add fast-drying concrete mix and water. Some blurt out, "Little more to the right, Mr. Keller. No left." Depending upon the child, we swap jobs, with them adding water and mix to the hole while I steady the post. The concrete mix hardens quickly and the post stands perfectly in position. Later we add cross bars to finish the main structure. We'll add the wire in Spring.

It is interesting to see how the nature of a novel task can influence the motivation of a child to work. Chores such as weeding often require lots of nudging and persuasion; it is a garden constant. But the kids jump in feet and arms first to dig a hole with an interesting tool and to work with concrete. During this project, not one child asks for the time or when was the session ending; they want to stay longer and finish the entire job even though it is exhausting.

OCTOBER OUTING: HUNT THE WILD MUSHROOM

Before the leaves cover the forest ground, a few wet days in late September or early October will cause an explosion of mushrooms. And even if you don't want to harvest them for food, they are a wonder to view with their delicate forms and colors.

One of the most spectacular, easy to identify and tasty is chicken-of-the-woods (Laetiporus sulphureus), a large, smooth mushroom that ranges in color from bright to yellowish orange. Oyster mushrooms (Pleurotus ostreatus) are also easy to spot. They look very similar to an oyster shell and are typically white or cream colored. But for every delicious mushroom there are death caps (Amanita phalloides) that will kill with a few ingested bites. If you decide to forage, be very careful and sure of your identifications.

STONE-HARD PUMPKINS

"I got a rock," was the continuous refrain of Charlie Brown as he looked to collect treats during Halloween. I feel somewhat like the giver of rocks to a group of Charlie Browns at the Harvest Festival at Ann's Place. My clients are attempting to carve some small sugar pumpkins (*Cucurbita pepo*) I brought as part of the activities, but with the first moves to cut into the gourds, knives bend against the hardness of the pumpkins.

"These knives aren't working," says Nina.

Perhaps the knives are to blame, but after having a go at Nina's pumpkin with the knife I'd given her, I determine that I purchased over a dozen rock-hard sugar pumpkins. I have since discovered that sugar pumpkins are not like your standard big orange gourd, soft and easy to cut with those cheap pumpkin knives you can get at the Dollar Store. Rather they are like acorn squash (*Cucurbita pepo* var. *turbinata*): hard to pierce with a knife but good eating once baked to a delicious, tender sweetness.

Like the survivors they all are, my clients take the difficulties in stride. Those who have the requisite strength and dexterity hollow out and cut faces into their pumpkins. Others decide to use felt-tip pens to sketch a face, waiting, perhaps, for a Sawzall or other appropriate power tool to later make their cuts. They enjoy the challenge.

"We'll be making mulling spices too," I say, turning away from the gourds and toward a table laid with spices. "What I would like each of you to do is smell the combined spices and then smell each spice individually. You should consider two things in making your mulling spice. The first is whether you smell each spice in the mix. The next is which individual spices you like and which ones you don't. Those preferences will help you make a better proportional mix."

Clients take turns grabbing the mulling spice jar holding cinnamon (*Cinnamomum verum*), allspice (*Pimenta dioica*), clove (*Syzygium aromaticum*), orange peel (*Citrus sinensis)*, lemon peel (*Citrus lemon*), nutmeg (*Myristica fragrans*), and cardamom (*Elettaria cardamomum*) and inhale deeply. They all like it, some to the point of wanting to clasp the jar to their face like a fragrant oxygen mask. But this is not the case once they sample individual spices.

"This is gross."

"I can't smell anything."

"I don't like this."

All misgivings evaporate as the warm mulled cider is served. Most ask for seconds. A few for thirds.

These comparisons help me to better understand clients' likes and dislikes. That is further driven home as I start to prepare dessert for the group and ask how many people want whipped cream with their apple (*Malus domestica*) pie or pumpkin (*Cucurbita*) bread I had baked that morning. Out of our group of nine, only four wanted this topping. I was surprised as my whipped cream usually has people fighting over the remnants in the bowl. What I didn't realize is that for varying reasons, many of my clients are lactose intolerant or they are vegan. Some are limited by their current cancer therapies while others prefer a healthier diet.

CALLED ON ACCOUNT OF SNOW

When I get home after working at the Meadow Ridge senior community, I hope to get some gardening done before the weather turns. Nothing special, just repotting and transplanting some of my greens into the cold frame. While driving home it begins to rain; it is the cold rain of Fall that chills you to the bone regardless of attire. Driving north, the precipitation starts to mix with light flurries. By the time I arrive home, there is already a light dusting of snow on the roof of my house and on leaves unaccustomed to this type of cover.

It is October. It is not supposed to snow. But you need to not only accept but expect the unusual in what Nature dishes out at any time of year. Instead of skeletons, I have plants full of leaves waiting to fully show off their Fall colors. It is supposed to be their time. But it isn't. They are coated in white.

For me the first snow of the year is often a reflective time as I remember the more youthful activities of sledding, snowball fights, and shoveling the driveway with my father. I also think of walking home from university with my wife when we were young students. In these memories, the snow covers a barren, dirty ground denuded of plant life. The snow purifies and, in a way, gives new life as light reflects off its veneer. It clothes naked trees and shrubs in white.

That is not the case today. Instead, the arrival of snow is ill timed, forcing leaves to abandon their perches prematurely. Hostas (*Hosta*), which should be dormant in the ground, are shivering under the weight of snow. The brilliant red leaves of our Japanese maple (*Acer palmatum*) are speckled and hanging low. Leaves too delicate to catch snow wave wildly about, not wanting to be trapped in an icy shawl. The only tree that seems at peace is our concolor fir (*Abies concolor*), which now appears Christmas-card perfect.

I don't worry that bulbs have not been planted, the water hose is still out, and all the gardening activities for Fall have been placed on hold. With the first snow, you consider the future of your garden and what you will do in the months ahead. Today, Fall has been deferred and my thoughts are focused upon my garden.

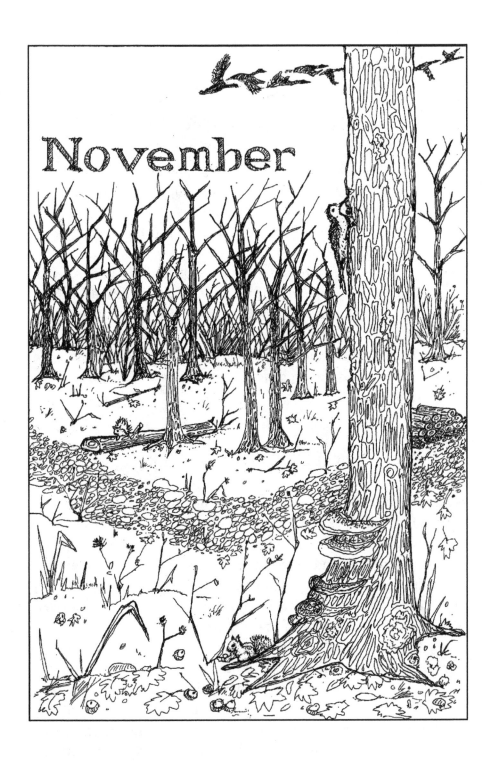

November

NOVEMBER: KILLING FROSTS

The frosty moon and cooling temperatures of November remove the remaining green from deciduous vegetation. The dark forests of Summer and early Fall are now light and airy with leafless trees revealing the sky.

Lawns have started to turn brown, and the weeds that were so troublesome months ago have retreated for the season. Squirrels, chipmunks, and other rodents collect the last remaining seeds to keep themselves fed during the long Winter ahead. Leaves need raking and garden beds require their final tidying up.

WEEDING OUT ANGER

My first realization that gardening has a therapeutic effect was in the early 1990s when I worked at a Stamford, Connecticut–based company called Gartner as an analyst. At Gartner I evaluated the technology products and services used by manufacturing companies to better their operations. My clients depended upon my counsel to help them decide which products and services to buy. Such purchases were typically in the millions of dollars. There was a lot of pressure.

By the end of the workday my nerves would be frayed and my disposition tense. Even a forty-five-minute drive home would not be enough to soothe the savage beast within, as decisions would be revisited and work would continue via cell-phone conference calls.

One of the ways I decompressed was to spend time in the garden even before seeing my wife and children. After pulling the car into the garage, I would look over the vegetables, pull a few weeds, and water plants in need of a drink. As I spent more time in the garden, the stress and pressure of the workday disappeared like so many dandelion (*Taraxacum officinale*) seeds blowing in the wind. Within twenty minutes, I was renewed.

I reflect on those days after I pick up Peter from his class. Head ducked low in his coat with his hands in pockets, he has a scowl on his freckled face. As we walk toward the Children's Garden, I ask Peter how he feels and how his week is progressing.

"I'm really pissed off," says Peter.

"What's the matter?"

"My friends are leaving and I hate it." Two of Peter's friends are leaving Green Chimneys and Peter is feeling alone and upset. He wants to hit something.

"Peter, I know how you feel. Friends have moved away from me too. But it's part of growing up and it'll happen again to you."

He nods but can't choke back a few tears.

Because Peter enjoys physical work, I decide to tackle a fairly hard, long-delayed weeding job where we need to pull large tufts of crabgrass (*Digitaria sanguinalis*), mint (*Mentha*), and other thickly rooted plants that reside against the fence near the gooseberry (*Ribes uva-crispa*) and raspberry (*Rubus idaeus*) patches. It is a physically exhausting job, as the roots will not give up their grasp on the soil easily even in November.

"Peter, try to transfer your pain and anger to the weeds. Every time you feel bad, send your feelings to the plant that's giving you a hard time. Trust me, it will make you feel better."

As Peter stands over the weeds, he delays any action as he looks past the meadow where our sheep graze against a backdrop of foothills occupied by leafless trees. He is zoned out.

"Come on, Peter. Put your back into it," I call out, trying to shock him out of complacency. "Get to work."

With that nudge, Peter looks up toward me and starts to work, at first slowly and then with more gusto. Soon he is digging, prying, and pulling up weeds, filling our wheelbarrow, taking a break only when it is full and needs to be emptied into the compost heap. He grabs a tuft of crabgrass and with all of his strength pulls back hard against it. He starts to liberate it from the ground with a little tear before a larger rip follows along with an explosion of soil. He flies backward landing on his bottom.

"Wow! Look at this, Mr. Keller!" he says, holding up a mass of still green weeds.

Other clumps are beyond his strength alone and together we pull the recalcitrant plants from the ground. His worries have evaporated, working next to me, smiling through the perspiration on his face. Before he knows it, our time is over; he is a sweaty mess and it is time to clean up.

"Are we done? Can't we keep going?" he asks.

"I'm sorry, Peter, but it's time to get you back to class. How do you feel?"

"Much better. That was great. Thank you."

We smile at our accomplishment: Much of the space is devoid of weeds. Before we leave the garden, Peter gets a piece of lemon leaf (*Rumex acetosa*) and some carrots (*Daucus carota* subsp. *sativus*) that are wintering over. He chomps down on his veggie reward, happy and content.

"Can we do this next week?" he asks.

"I'm sure we can, Peter. There will always be weeds to pull."

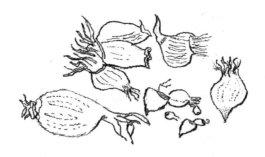

FLOWERS AND FOOD

In almost every exercise with clients, there is always something that they take back home with them that is made in class. But the elderly who live at Meadow Ridge, a senior community, often do not have the capability to bring class projects back with them. Those in wheelchairs or using walkers face even more challenges, which I must consider in organizing any activity.

"Today we're going to pot up food and flowers. Each of you will be able to take back a couple of pots to place outside your apartments. In Spring you'll get flowers and food from your plantings."

I then upend a paper bag on the table, spilling out a wide variety of bulbs and passing them around for my clients to identify. The gardeners in the group are quick to speak:

"Daffodil (*Narcissus*)."

"Crocus (*Crocus*)."

"Muscari (*Muscari armeniacum*)."

Then Gladys asks, "What is a garlic (*Allium sativum*) doing here?"

I reply, "That's the food part. Each of you can create an arrangement of bulbs for display as well as a separate one to grow fresh garlic."

With that I separate a German red garlic head into its individual teeth and pass them around. "Take a sniff and let me know what you think." German red is one of my favorite garlic types as it has very pungent and flavorful characteristics. My clients love it.

Rena talks about how she used to chop up garlic to make her mother's spaghetti sauce. "My hands always smelled but that was how I knew I was doing it right. Mother never did give me a formal recipe."

Before class I placed buckets of soil in the middle of the tables with pitchers of water next to them. "You will get dirty now, as we need to mix the soil with water. When ready, it should be moist enough to form a ball without water dripping when you squeeze it."

The response is mixed. Some dig in with both hands to mix the water and the soil enthusiastically. Others less desirous of getting their hands dirty opt to use a trowel. Sally, who has arthritis, loves squeezing the warm soil with her gnarled fingers while another person adds water. Her hands, now coated with soil, stir up earthy scents as she works it slowly in a repetitive fashion.

"It's been so long since I have touched soil. It's wonderful," Sally says as she pulls her muddy hands from the bucket.

I then instruct the group how to plant and layer the bulbs in the pots so they will emerge at the right times and how to organize them to produce the best visual effect. This kicks off lots of discussion about gardens of the past and their former homes.

"Can I leave these inside when I'm done?" asks Janice.

"No, they need to be chilled to set and then bloom. It's perfect to leave them out on your balcony for Winter."

"Is it any different for the garlic?"

"No, and they won't be ready for harvest until late June or early July. But you'll get garlic scapes to harvest and use for cooking before the bulb is mature."

Only half of my clients pot up garlic, since many of them no longer cook. Most are able to return to their apartments without help, though not Sally, who potted up daffodils and garlic but is unable to take her pots with her. I carry them and walk next to Sally as she slowly makes her way to her apartment.

As we enter her apartment, I see a vase of faded flowers that need to be discarded on an end table near the entrance. After I throw them out and clean the vase, I place the pots on her balcony in a nook that is sheltered from the wind. Sally thanks me for the help and sits in an easy chair looking out the sliding glass doors at the pots, imagining the flowers that will emerge next Spring.

RAKING MEMORIES AND LEAVES

I haven't raked leaves at my mother's house on Long Island for quite a few decades. The yard service made a final lawn cut and visit a few weeks back, but since then it seems as if all the neighboring trees decided to deliver their leaves to my mother's lawn for the season. Her trees—all oaks (*Quercus*)—have been hanging onto their leaves stubbornly, not wanting to give up this year's production. It was as if they decided that this was the season to wear a raccoon coat of dried, brittle brown foliage; no rain or wind will remove a single leaf.

Looking upward at the future blanket for my mother's lawn, I know that I need to remove the neighbors' leaves. In the garage there is a pile of old plastic bags and an even older rake missing a few teeth that my father used years ago before he turned over that duty to others. I ask my mother to join me outside. To my surprise she does.

The straw-like zoysia (*Zoysia japonica*) grass is holding onto the leaves with more vigor than does my fescue (*Festuca arundinacea*) at home. Perhaps it doesn't realize that the trees above will deposit yet another insulator. Regardless, I rake the leaves into large dumpling-shaped piles in the middle of the lawn. It is time to bag.

My mother walks over to take a look and I ask her if she would like to jump into a pile. She laughs and says that was my pleasure from years ago. I think back and remember that the piles seemed so much larger then. My father and I would rake leaves into a heap as tall as I was, and then I would burrow inside like a creature preparing to hibernate for the season. It was warm inside, and there was an unmistakable sour-sweet smell of decay.

I tower over the leaf piles now, not wanting to jump in but to bag them for the town service to haul away to compost. At my home, I rake the leaves into the backyard woods. But in my mother's manicured neighborhood, there is no such space and everything must be removed.

I open a bag, shake it out, and place it on the ground, anchoring it with my feet and holding an edge while my other arm pulls swaths of leaves into the bag. Like a piston, my arm rhythmically sweeps the area until I need to stop and rebuild the pile. Pulling the bag off the ground, I shake it and then punch the leaves down, compacting them into a tight mass before repeating the exercise. My father taught this technique to me.

My mother is supervising the operation from the front step, sitting down carefully as she places her cane next to her and a piece of cardboard under her backside as a cushion. I walk over during a break sitting next to her, and we reminisce about how my father used to feed the squirrels with walnuts from his hand. He would squat down in an impossibly balanced configuration with his knees high and his bottom low, rhythmically bouncing while he would smack the walnuts (*Juglans*) or filberts (*Corylus maxima*) together with both hands, announcing his arrival.

Initially cautious, the squirrels took to my father (and his nuts) quickly. But they soon came to expect his attention on a consistent basis. If they perceived he was late for a feeding they would come to the house, congregate on the stoop, and chastise my father that he was late and needed to come outside. And in a Pavlovian manner my father would respond.

My mother and I laugh. I hand her an acorn and go back to work.

NOVEMBER CRAFT: START AMARYLLIS AND PAPERWHITE BULBS

*Amaryllis (*Hippeastrum*) and paperwhite (*Narcissus papyraceus*) bulbs have arrived in barrels at nurseries and big box stores. Some are in cartons holding plastic pots and growing medium. Each takes four to six weeks to flower, so if you desire to use them as a decorative accent for the holidays, mid to late November is the best time to start them.*

Paperwhites come in one type: white and fragrant. To some, their overly sweet smell is unpleasant. Amaryllises, on the other hand, have little smell but come in countless varieties—large, small, single, multiflowered, solid, striped, even multicolored— making it difficult to choose. Do yourself a favor and pick a bunch.

FINAL HARVESTS

The harvests are getting leaner in the Children's Garden as the sun and temperatures continue to drop. We still have carrots, lettuce (*Lactuca sativa*), radishes (*Raphanus sativus*), Swiss chard (*Beta vulgaris* subsp. *vulgaris*), and collard greens (*Brassica oleracea* var. *acephala*). We planted this row in late August, and we are into our second harvest of the season for the greens. An additional batch of lettuce is ready to pick as are the radishes. The radishes are the French breakfast variety, which has a shape that is unfamiliar to most of the children. Mary, who is pulling the radishes, is confused by their cylindrical profile and red-and-white color.

"That can't be a radish. Radishes are round and all red."

"Some are like that. But like people and animals, they come in all different shapes and colors."

"No way!"

"Way! Many radishes are red and round, but there are white ones, purple ones, and pink ones. Some are round and some are long like a carrot." Mary hopes that we can grow some of these other varieties next year. I tell her that I will try to get some purple radishes in the ground for next season.

At the same time we do a second cutting of the lettuce. Picking lettuce is more difficult than radishes as we want to preserve the roots to get additional harvests. When we harvest lettuce I ask the children to cut it at least an inch above the ground. Many have a difficult time being that precise and often either cut the plant too low or pull out an entire plant. As Luis pulls out a couple of lettuce plants, he asks why it matters.

"You may not realize it, but lettuce can grow back like grass after cutting it," I say. "If we pull out the entire plant we will get only one harvest. This way we can get two or three."

Luis understands but has impulse control challenges. It is difficult for him to manage his emotions so that the plants remain undamaged. We move to a different activity.

The collard greens and the Swiss chard will still need a little longer to reach harvest size. I'm not sure if the carrots will be ready next month, but if they aren't I'll just leave them in the ground to harvest in March or April. The Agribon hoop house we built over the row has helped all the vegetables grow and survive the nightly frosts. Some of the kids are wondering what we are doing in the garden this late in the season. I can't wait to bring them back in December. Perhaps there will be snow.

SPREADING SEEDS

While plants go dormant, or die in the case of annuals, there is still plenty of life in the garden. One of the more animated examples now is the birds that are either passing through during their migration or have decided to stay and tough it out for the season. To attract them, however, nourishment is needed. While my yard holds many bird-attracting plants including winterberry (*Ilex verticillata*), crabapple (*Malus*), Japanese beautyberry (*Callicarpa japonica*), chokecherry (*Prunus virginiana*), and cranberry viburnum (*Viburnum opulus* var. *americanum*), they are not enough by themselves to feed the flocks that visit our house for the entire Winter. Feeders are needed to supplement what is available in my garden.

I have been gathering materials over the past few months to build bird feeders as a project for my Ann's Place clients, who now are gathered around a large table. Awaiting instruction, they look puzzled as our collection of materials must appear a little strange: wire, knives, jars of peanut butter, dishes of bird seed and piles of pine (*Pinus*) and spruce (*Picea*) cones.

"We'll be making feeders that can attract most of the birds that winter in the Northeast," I start. "The seeds will attract blue jays, finches, juncos, also known as snowbirds, and many others. The peanut butter will attract woodpeckers and other birds that like lots of fat."

I show them a finished feeder and they start to smile. It is a pine cone coated with peanut butter and covered with seeds. "You need to smear a good amount of peanut butter into the cracks of the cones and then roll them in the seeds in front of you. That makes the feeder," I say. "But don't forget to put on the wire first or you'll get your hands quite messy. Make as many as you can."

And with these simple instructions the class goes to work. It is not as easy as one might believe to fill the crevices of a cone with peanut butter so seeds are able to stick to it. Some try smearing on a very thin layer, which when rolled produces a feeder without many seeds. Questions start coming:

"How can I stop the squirrels from eating this?"

"Will this attract a cardinal?"

"Can I reuse the cone when the birds clean it off?"

"How long will it last?"

I try my best to answer these questions, but in many cases I tell them it is something that they will need to discover for themselves. They nod their heads in acknowledgment and continue to spread the gooey paste on more cones that will become seasonal decoration for their yard and food for some nearby creature.

NOVEMBER OUTING: TAKE STOCK OF THE GARDEN

The garden is nearly spent. Seed heads remind us of the beautiful plants and flowers of months past. But the barren nature of the landscape gives us pause and time to reflect on the architecture of our plantings.

Did some plants disappoint, become spent, or do badly? Are there new opportunities to expand certain spaces? Did you discover a new plant that you want to use in the garden? Walk around the garden and envision how next year can look and make plans to effect the needed changes.

NOVEMBER BOUQUETS

With Thanksgiving a few days away, I continue to scurry in the garden to finish all my chores before the snows hit. Given the spate of warm weather we have had this Fall, this urgency may be the result of experience borne from years when snow has covered the ground from Thanksgiving to mid April. You never know when it is going to start. I bring Charlotte along to help me as she is always willing and enjoys her time outside with me.

Today's chore is to cut back all the remaining irises (*Iris*), lilies (*Lilium*), hostas (*Hosta*), and other plants that are on their way out or close to it. Cutting back some of the Montauk daisies (*Nipponanthemum nipponicum*), I notice that some of their blooms are still fresh on the stem. Charlotte helps me choose the ones with the most viable flowers. She gathers them in her hands to make two bouquets: one for her mother and one for her grandmother. Charlotte suggests that we look for other flowers to accompany the tiny bouquets she has in her hands. We discover more flowers than I would have thought possible.

Ironically most of the chrysanthemums (*Chrysanthemum*) that we bought a few months back have already bloomed and died. While they are sold as perennials, the mums from local nurseries are often annuals with short-lived flowers, though they are lush and full in their prime. Montauk daisies, on the other hand, are hardy and will winter over for many years. Their blooms may not be as extravagant as garden-variety mums, but they are dependable.

Walking around the side of the house, Charlotte spots Shasta daisies (*Leucanthemum superbum*) that are still sporting blooms. I cut a few of them, giving them to Charlotte to organize. With this type of luck, Charlotte and I decide to take a more expansive stroll to see what else we can find.

A yellow butterfly bush (*Buddleia davidii)* I planted a few years ago is still full of bright yellow plumes, some of which I cut. Next to that bush, a purple butterfly bush has long since gone to seed, but the delicate texture of its cone-like seed spires gives them a life that I think will look well in a vase.

Charlotte points out the flowers on the rose (*Rosa*) bushes: One of our shrubs has a spray of tiny pink roses, perfect for the bouquets. I snip just what we need, leaving developing buds in the unrealistic hope that I will be able to pick their flowers this December.

All the obvious flowers have been picked so we start to seek unusual elements for the bouquets. I find a specimen in our winterberry, which has long since dropped its leaves but is full of fat red berries. The winterberry is a holly, one of the few that are deciduous, and to the untrained eye it can easily be confused with a viburnum (*Viburnum*) this time of year. The berries stand in sharp distinction against its gray bark; their shape and color will add a nice contrast to the other plants Charlotte and I have picked.

The last flower is a surprise as neither I nor my wife planted it. Yellow corydalis (*Corydalis lutea*) has flowered in delicate trumpet-like, yellow clusters. It will fill in the bouquets' open spaces nicely. Charlotte tucks it into place and we head back for the warmth of our house.

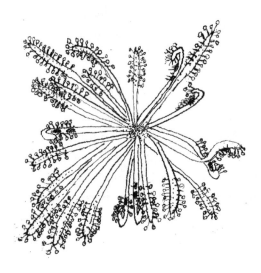

FEED ME KRELBORN, FEED ME NOW!

Whenever I start working with a child in the Children's Garden, there is often a mutual sizing up. I evaluate the child to determine the best course of therapy. The child, in turn, looks me over to determine what type of person I am and if I am worth their effort or share any common interests. And sometimes I have been able find a particular interest and use it to motivate.

For instance, when a slot opened up for a new student, Tracy said that Seymour would be a good match for me but I should stay alert because he is obsessed with carnivorous plants. For me this is a serendipitous coupling since I propagate them as a hobby. A few months ago, I brought a variety of these plants to school for the students to look at and examine.

I fell in love with Nature's own bug zappers when I vacationed in California for a wedding years ago and had the opportunity to visit the California Carnivores nursery, which specializes in these unusual meat eaters. After reading the owner's book, *The Savage Garden*, I was hooked.

When I meet Seymour the first time, it takes all of three minutes before he starts to tell me that he wants to work in the garden with carnivorous plants and asks do I know anything about them.

"We don't have any carnivorous plants here at Green Chimneys. But yes, Seymour, I know a lot about carnivorous plants. In fact, I grow them."

With that his eyes open wide and he wants to talk about nothing except carnivorous plants. We chat for about ten minutes and then I tell him that we need to go to work.

"But I don't want to work. I want to talk about carnivorous plants with you."

"I'll make a deal with you, Seymour. If you work well with me, follow directions, and do your job, I'll give you a carnivorous plant after Thanksgiving."

His eyes open wide again. "My own plant? But how will I take care of it?"

"I'll teach you, and I'll give you a plant that is easy to take care of. You can have a Cape sundew (*Drosera capensis*)."

Cape sundews are like weeds as they self-seed with abandon. I started out with one a year ago and now have over a dozen. They have become a favorite of my wife in the kitchen as their little leaves have sticky orbs of mucilage that trap and consume insects. Since they have made a home in our kitchen, it is nearly devoid of bugs. And when well fed they grow quickly: The sundews in the kitchen went from seed to the size of my fist within a year. I believe Seymour will have similar success.

With that motivation, Seymour becomes the perfect student. Everything we work on together he does with enthusiasm and care. He wants to talk a lot about different types of carnivorous plants, and when we have an opportunity we do. Before Thanksgiving, I start to teach him about how a carnivorous plant needs to be watered with either distilled or rain water and be kept moist in a water tray. I tell him about their temperature requirements: Cape sundews are warm-weather plants that do not require dormancy, whereas Venus fly traps (*Dionaea muscipula*) and North American pitcher plants (*Sarracenia*) do require a cold-weather dormant period. These discussions are just a prelude to the lesson of the day, which he always picks up very quickly.

Every day I'm with Seymour, he talks about getting his plant and tells me how good a job he plans to do that day. Even when he is moody and does not want to work, the thought of getting his own plant motivates him enough so that he gets on with the job and is successful.

The week after Thanksgiving I make good on my promise: Seymour gets his Cape sundew. It is small but healthy with tiny drops of mucilage on its tips. In the angled light, they appear as little jewels arranged in a floret. A few gnats have made the mistake of getting too close and are being consumed slowly.

"I am going to be away for Christmas. Won't it die from not being watered?" asks Seymour.

"Just leave it in a nice container of distilled or rain water and it will be fine for the days you are gone," I reply.

He smiles and takes his plant to show his friends.

To keep him motivated I promise to teach him how to propagate Venus fly traps this Spring when they emerge from dormancy. That's the plant he really wants.

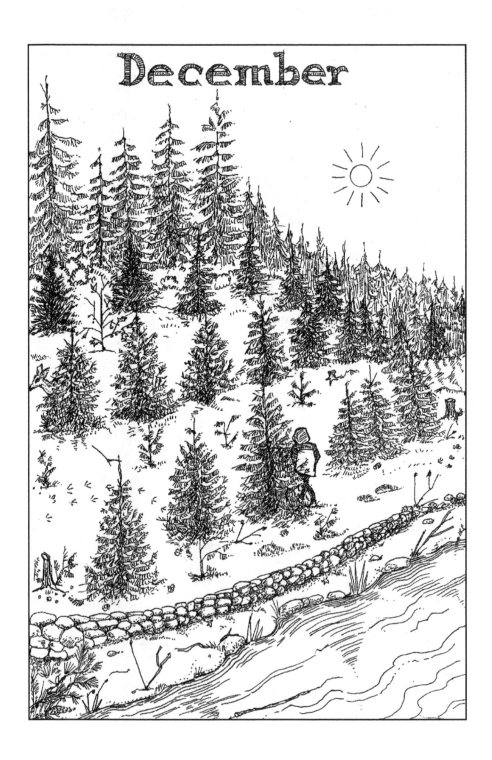

December

DECEMBER: READYING FOR WINTER

The beds have been cleaned, the bulbs planted, the flowers have faded, and the garden is desolate. After a mild November, the tiny yellow flowers of witch hazel (Hamamelis virginiana) *are persisting, but most everything else has long since become dormant.*

Seed heads of our coneflowers (Echinacea) *stand alone, waiting to be eaten by hungry birds. The grass has faded to a light straw hue with only evergreens and a few dried fruits and berries enlivening the landscape with some color. But a few chores linger.*

FLOWER POWER

As life in the garden winds down, cleaning old beds and pulling dead or dying plants takes priority. That is the case in the first few days of December when we must pull cosmos *(Cosmos bipinnatus)* from one of the beds near the Green Chimneys administration building.

It seems wrong to remove these tall sentinels as some are still in full bloom while others have some buds. I tell a couple of aides and teachers that I will be pulling the plants today and they are more than welcome to make as many bouquets from the flowers as they can. "That's great," says Anika, a teacher. "It's my favorite flower." Over coffee this morning, Anika was a little morose, but the prospect of a colorful bunch of posies perks her right up.

My students are excited that they can pull these plants from the soil. They line up to yank a bunch of four-to-six-foot stems. They position each foot on the side of a clump of stems they gather together by hand. With a hard tug, a slow tearing sound accompanies the liberation of the roots from the soil. Some of the root masses need extra persuasion in the form of a shovel or a helper, as their grip on the soil is too much for a single child to overcome.

"By the way, Alejandro, after you finish pulling plants, you can make a bouquet of flowers if you would like," I say to one of the day's first weeders. Alejandro loves that idea and works even harder than he had been before. After he pulls the cosmos from the soil, he places them carefully so it will be easy to cull the flowers.

Clearing the cosmos is also grabbing attention from passers by. Pedestrians shoot over looks of puzzlement, disdain, and sadness at what we are doing in the cosmos beds. To allay their concerns, I have my students offer everyone who walks by a flower or two. This becomes a new job that the students share during our sessions. Nearly every time a flower is offered, our working group gets a big smile and thanks from those who accept one. Janet, a social worker with whom I had worked previously says, "This is wonderful. You have made my day."

Cleaning up these beds at the end of the season is a big job, so I spend most of my time in the beds pulling cosmos and giving flowers to strangers, young and old. As we broadcast the seed heads of spent flowers into the bed, a few observers inquire what we are doing. I stop my pulling and get out my pocket knife and cut a blossom, a blooming flower, and a dried-up seed pod. Using these three examples I explain to them and my students the life cycle of a cosmos and how it reproduces. Most are intrigued and thank me after they select a flower or two to take away.

In the 1980s I worked in New York City and took the Long Island Railroad home each evening. I would often buy flowers sold by followers of Rev. Sun Myung Moon, who founded the Unification Church, as I neared Penn Station. Unlike those followers, mine have no agenda. They just want to give a flower to someone to make them happy.

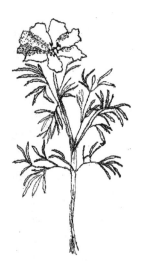

A SMELLY START

When I begin a horticultural-therapy session, I attempt to break the ice with something unexpected. It can be some freshly picked berries from nearby bushes that the birds and animals have missed or slug-free greens that I just pulled from my garden. This time of year, however, such pickings are quite slim. When I arrive for my class at Ann's Place, I hope to harvest some herbs that have outlasted the snow and recent twenty-degree nights.

When I start to clip some American holly (*Ilex opaca*) branches, I am pleasantly surprised by the fact that the Cleveland sage (*Salvia clevelandii*) has a few branches that are intact with green shoots. Some of the lavender *(Lavandula angustifolia)* is still blue green and our mountain mint *(Pycnanthemum muticum)* is beginning to send out a second or third growth from its root ball. I clip these offerings and bring them in.

Delivering something different to clients before we start a session opens their senses to creativity and possibilities that they often have not considered before walking into the room, particularly as Winter approaches. And using the sense of smell can be a very powerful way to remember forgotten events and experiences.

I pass out stems to each individual, asking them to both identify and tell the group if they like them or not. At first, scents are nuanced and difficult to discern. Few clients are familiar with the best way to express the fragrance of the herbs by rubbing the leaves and then smelling their fingers. Once I clue in the group to this trick, slight scents become powerful fragrances.

"Oh my god! This is horrible," says Lisa about the sage.

"This is quite relaxing," says Kristin of the lavender.

"I think this is a mint," says Marie, not sure of its type.

The sage, in particular, produces a very powerful scent when rubbed. Few are neutral about it, and it is either love or hate. But one client lingers over each branch. She approaches each leaf carefully, inhaling deeply with each rubbing. She is wearing a kerchief over her head, indicating that she has little if any hair. Her face is thin and pale.

"I can't believe this! This is the first time in a year that I have been able to smell anything. This is wonderful!" says Naia, exhaling with pleasure. A small tear emerges from her right eye as a smile comes to her face. Other clients quietly watch her and absorb some of the pure joy she exudes.

DECEMBER CRAFT: MAKE ORNAMENTS AND DECORATIONS

Seasonal celebrations are enhanced by creating handmade ornaments that use Nature's castoffs. Tiny three-inch-wide logs can be cut into slices and decorated by hand to be hung around the house. Acorns can be fashioned into a wide variety of creatures and knickknacks.

Transform conifer cones into elves, deer, and other creatures that please the eye. Holly (Ilex aquifolium) and other berries can be draped on mantles and tables around beloved pictures and memorabilia. Moss (Bryophyta) can be collected from rocks and walls to form a lush and living carpet that will hold and accentuate anything resting upon it. There is much to gather: You just need to keep an eye peeled, ready for inspiration.

UNEXPECTED CONSEQUENCES

December is a challenging month to teach in the Children's Garden. Harvesting vegetables and fruits is mostly over, weeds are in abeyance, planting is in the past, and clean-up is complete. This is the time to be innovative in horticultural therapy, to come up with projects that will both teach and excite. I am able to try something atypical for December as the temperature hits the fifties and the sun is shining.

This is the perfect day to take my students around the grounds on a scavenger hunt. In this exercise, each child gets a clipboard with a piece of paper headed, "Finding Flora: Things in the Garden," and the letters of the alphabet split into two columns, providing twenty-six possibilities in total.

"Flora is the goddess of flowers according to Roman mythology. She is more appropriately associated with Spring, but we can search around the garden for her influence. The goal is to find something, preferably a plant, for all letters A to Z," I tell my students.

This class hits all the different types of goals we have in horticultural therapy. It is good exercise as we spend an hour walking around the campus and bending over to examine different aspects of Nature; it also helps students manage small motor skills through writing on a clipboard. It facilitates social interaction as conversation flows freely; I find that with these types of exercises children often let down their guard and confide in you. It helps them emotionally as a walk in the garden often has a calming effect. And finally, it forces them to use their minds. Once you find "grass" for the letter G, finding "garlic" or "goat" doesn't count; you also have to spell and examine Nature with an open mind.

Because the community of children I work with is very diverse, I expect to get a wide range of responses. But in this case, I am thrown for a loop as each of my students reacts in a very different way than I anticipate.

I don't expect much enthusiasm from my first child of the day. Adam is a quiet and melancholy boy. I grab a clipboard and we start to find and account for different types of plants. He somewhat responds with interest, writing names and checking letters as I hope.

Within a few minutes, however, he asks if we can go to the wildlife pens to see the birds of prey, including owls, turkey vultures, bald eagles, and a condor.

"Not a problem, Adam. In fact, I thought that we would need to go there to fill out our list."

Adam immediately brightens up and becomes very focused on the task at hand, combing the garden and surrounding areas for different plants and animals to fill in his sheet. At the end of the hour he gets twenty-four out of the twenty-six letters, missing only Q and Z. I take him back to his class as a happy child.

The next student, Demetrius, is very bright and always enthusiastic about working in the garden regardless of the task. He looks for praise constantly and will work hard to obtain it. I anticipate that for him the scavenger hunt will be a great treat. But when I tell him what we will be doing, he gives me a hard look.

"Why am I doing this? This sounds stupid. This is not a job."

I am taken aback. This type of rebuke is not something I expect, particularly from Demetrius. "This is a job," I say. "It's an exercise that will help you better understand what is in the garden."

"No it's not. It's not a job. You're making me do this because I suck," he says, becoming increasingly agitated.

"No, no, that's not it at all. Think of this as training," I say. "When you have a real job, there are days that you have to go for training to learn a new skill or refresh an old one. You should think of this in the same way as it will help you remember and identify all the different plants we have in the garden and organize them in your mind."

Demetrius thinks about this for a moment and then says, "Well, I understand but still don't think it's a real job. I guess I'll try."

"Good, Demetrius, and next week we'll be harvesting some of the Swiss chard and lettuce in the garden."

He looks around the garden indifferently and in thirty minutes gets eighteen letters.

My next child, Shelly, does not embrace the exercise. Like Demetrius, she doesn't think it is a real job and is sullen during our entire time together, not paying attention or even trying. She finds nine letters, though she surprises me by spelling asparagus (*Asparagus officinalis*) and strawberry (*Fragaria ×ananassa*) correctly. After our exercise she complains to teachers and others that I am a poor teacher. It takes a couple weeks of closely working with her to return to Shelly's good graces.

The day's experiences puzzle me. A prior group of students in Spring had loved the exercise. This day I was successful with one child but others saw the task as a punishment. Perhaps it is the change of venue that is the issue, walking the grounds rather than staying in the garden; children in this facility don't like to be surprised with an altered routine. When they work with me, a typical job is to dig in the garden, pull weeds, or transplant seedlings; it is a physical challenge. It is unusual to hold a pen and pad and think about plants. Perhaps they associated this scavenger hunt with schoolwork, which they want to escape when they are in the garden. I'm not sure, but when I try this again perhaps I will need to better explain and sell the activity to my students.

DECEMBER OUTING: COLLECT OUTDOOR MATERIALS FOR DRIED BOUQUETS

Bouquets gathered outdoors are often thought of as something we collect in Spring and Summer. But dried flowers, grasses, and other plants can make interesting combinations in the cooler months.

One of the showiest dried heads is that of hydrangea (Hydrangea), with its large, bulbous flowers sitting on an otherwise desiccated stem. Certain grasses such as sea oats (Uniola paniculata) have a lovely wavy form and hold their seeds throughout Winter. Garnished with the red berries of the winterberry (Ilex verticillata) or purple Japanese *beautyberry (*Callicarpa japonica*), a colorful and lasting bouquet can be gathered during a quick stroll.*

MOM ON ICE

An ice storm arrived the other day and it has been unusual in its persistence. Typically, when such weather events occur, we receive a slight layer of ice that disappears as quickly as it forms around branches, along walks, and on fencing. But an unusual chill is causing this quarter-inch-plus coating of ice to remain for days, affording me time to appreciate its beauty.

Everything on the ground is covered in an undulating sheet that crackles intermittently, sounding like dry cereal crunching in your mouth as I walk upon it. But no footprints remain behind me. The pointy, crystal-green blades of grass continue to stand firm as would stalagmites in an underground cavern.

Once the streets and my driveway are clear, Juana and I drive over to see my mother at Ridge Crest, a nursing home at the Meadow Ridge senior community. We arrive just before lunch time and she is just getting ready for the day. She gives us a big smile as the nursing aide combs her gray hair, making it neat.

"I didn't expect you today," she says. "What a wonderful surprise!"

"We would have come yesterday but the ice storm kept us at home," I reply.

"What ice storm?"

Juana and I point to the window in her room letting her see the rhododendrons (*Rhododendron*) sagging under the weight of ice. Beyond is a white lawn that shimmers as the sun reflects on the icy crystals embedded on the surface. I can tell that my mother would like to see more.

Comfortable in her wheelchair, with a red plaid wool lap blanket keeping her warm, we wheel her out of the nursing area toward a hallway with large windows and a view of trees and bushes. Stopping in front of a glass double door, my mother is in awe. A weeping cherry (*Prunus pendula*) has become a drooping crystalline figure with tiny shards of ice beneath it. A row of black chokeberries (*Aronia melanocarpa*) is topped with ice while a nearby crabapple tree (*Malus*) displays pendulous fruits encased in ice, looking like tiny, jeweled, red teardrops.

"It's so beautiful. I've never seen anything like it," says my mother. We sit and watch the light play with the plants. My mother doesn't want to leave the area, as the sparkling garden has her enthralled. Birds try to perch on the icy limbs of a nearby flowering dogwood (*Cornus florida*). One comically slips off a branch a few times before it is able to get a firm grip. Pieces of fallen ice are scattered over the lawn, appearing as sparkling albeit transitory diamonds.

We eventually arrive at the atrium, filled with tropical plants, whose three-story-high, translucent ceiling is covered with ice. Suddenly, without warning, sheets of ice slide downward sounding like marbles bouncing on the floor. Initially worried, my mother is calmed when we point out to her what is happening. She looks upward and then she sees for herself the ice move.

Next to her wheelchair, a small indoor waterfall splashes into a pond holding ornamental carp. The air is thick with humidity as the trees and undergrowth pump out oxygen. She takes in a deep breath and a smile comes to her face.

"Can we have a cup of tea?" asks my mother. "You bet," I reply, heading off to fulfill her request. As I fill a cup for her I look back and see her with her head tilted toward the sky, watching and listening for the ice to fall.

(This was one of the last times I saw my mother alive before she succumbed to COVID-19 in Spring.)

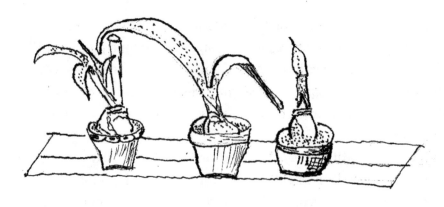

LATE LESSONS

One of the simpler horticultural therapy exercises is potting up: taking seeds, bulbs, or plants and putting them into a container. The trouble with this exercise, however, is that it can get boring and repetitive for clients, so you need an adjunct activity to spice it up. With this in mind I purchase ribbons, fabrics, foils, and other tchotchkes to decorate the plain plastic pots I have on hand. And since it is around the holidays, I clip two different types of holly that we have growing around the building as a last-minute decorative thought.

This class at Ann's Place has been nearly a year in the making as I was able to purchase eighteen amaryllis (*Hippeastrum*) bulbs for a dollar each, down from nine dollars, last January from a local supermarket. I thought that they would keep if I wrapped them in newspaper and left them in my unheated basement. I checked them during the year, and other than a whitening of some of the early leaves, they are solid and firm prior to class. I also went to a local nursery two months ago to purchase some leftover bulbs and placed them to chill in a bucket outside.

An extra bonus came in leftover bulbs I was able to obtain from a charity holiday sale at Ann's Place, so everyone can get a pot of paperwhites (*Narcissus papyraceus*) in addition to the bulbs I had already purchased. And as if on cue, everyone shows up ready to pot.

"With the exception of the paperwhites, all of these bulbs will give you flowers in the next few months. And they can be used later, either outside or inside, for years to come." I then explain the few things people need to do to pot up the bulbs. I have a good mix that will let people create different arrangements, some to start growing now and others to be left outside as they still need at least eight weeks of cold to set. There isn't much to say, so I place a big bin of soil in the center of the tables, get out the different bulbs, and tell my clients to get planting.

To my surprise nobody finds it boring; rather, they jump at the opportunity and the many different choices they have to consider. The table is a whirl of activity with everyone enjoying the chance to get their hands dirty in the mucky soil. As it turns out, the decorations I supplied are not that desired or needed, though the box of holly I cut is emptied. Clients wrap the pots with foil to ensure water will not drip out when they are transported back home.

I thought we might have too many bulbs, but each client pots up three containers with interesting mixes. A group of clients are happy to stay late to help me pot up twenty paperwhite and amaryllis containers for clients who are unable to attend the class. There are a few bulbs left over that I will take home for Juana.

After cleaning up, I am about to walk out the door when a client approaches. I know there are no more activities today.

"Pardon me, can I help you?" I ask.

"Yes, I'm here for horticultural therapy."

I tell her that the class was at 4:30, not now at 6:30. Her face falls and she gives off a tiny sigh. She starts to turn around to leave.

"Don't go. We can have a class, just you and me."

She looks at me, puzzled.

"But class is over, right?"

"It's okay. Let's get you some bulbs." I retrieve the bulbs that I had planned to give to Juana.

She removes her coat and hat, revealing stubble instead of a head of hair. I put down a plastic tablecloth with yellow flowers to protect the underlying craft paper. I get a container of soil, some pots and the remaining bulbs. We are ready. A small but growing smile emerges.

After giving her an amaryllis, I ask her if she wants to pot up some paperwhites as well as other bulbs. "Oh yes. That would be wonderful," she says, her voice cracking.

We pot up more bulbs and decorate them with a few sprigs of the holly. I tell her about the life cycles of bulbs and how she can care for them in the months to come. She relaxes as we chat, her hands sinking into the soil and manipulating the bulbs into place. She leaves our private session with pots of bulbs happy and peaceful.

Potting up is often derided in horticultural therapy as a "last resort" type of therapy. In this case, however, all the clients embraced the ability to feel and be one with the Earth; it is something that most folks have not done in a while. This different environment lets them relax and look forward to when the flowers will bloom in the months to come, bringing fresh scents in the middle of another Winter.

CHILLING GREENS

As Christmas nears, the garden still offers tasty treats, but few of my students accept such a proposition as nearly half a foot of snow dropped on us yesterday. Regardless, we still need to check the row hoop houses at the Children's Garden, remove the snow, and repair any damage. Before picking up my first student, I take a look at the garden: Some hoop houses that are sheltering our late-season crops have collapsed entirely, others partially, and a few are holding up well under the snow. Repairing the damage will be a challenge for some of my students.

The prior week in the garden was sunny, warm, and unseasonable. Today is sunny and slightly above freezing, but with the sun out, it is warming up fast. One of the challenges in working with children outside this time of year is to ensure that they keep warm while doing their jobs. A spare hat and pair of gloves is at the ready in the shed in case a student comes unprepared, which is the case more often than not. I pick up Enrique and we head toward the garden. He is surprised.

"Why are we going out? Everything has to be dead because of the snow," he says. "I'm cold."

"Why do you think that, Enrique?" I ask. He replies that it's Winter and everything has to be dead, especially under the snow. I tell him that he should hold his verdict on that until we finish our job this morning and that I have a hat and gloves for him. He shrugs.

After prying open the garden gate that is stuck in the snow, Enrique and I trudge our way toward the snow-covered hoop houses. One of the most damaged is framed with heavy-duty wire mesh because we had run out of the more sturdy PVC piping to support the Agribon fabric. The mesh had worked well so far, even in high winds, but five inches of snow and then a cold rain put too much weight upon it. It collapsed in the middle, looking like a squashed letter M. We need to shovel out the snow and fix the frame.

I hand a shovel and a pair of gloves to Enrique. "I don't know how to shovel snow," he says.

"We need to be careful," I say. "Take your shovel and turn it on its side so that it's like a knife. Gently cut the snow and then turn your shovel to pick up the chunk of snow that separates out. But you have to be careful so we don't rip the cloth that's covering the plants. Watch me."

I then demonstrate how to remove the snow. It takes Enrique a while to get the hang of it, but he is taking his time and is careful not to rip the cloth. As the snow separates into packed chunks, we play a game to see who can cut the largest piece. Enrique wins.

We soon remove all the snow and pull back the Agribon cloth and wire to reveal a thriving crop of winter lettuce *(Lactuca sativa)*. It is a little droopy but still in good shape. "How is that possible?" says Enrique with a shocked voice.

"It's possible, Enrique, because we put a blanket over the lettuce to keep it warm, just like the coat you're wearing is keeping you warm. How do you think you'd feel now if you didn't have a coat on?"

"Cold," he says.

"Right, so we need to put the blanket back on the lettuce to let it warm up." It is fairly early in the morning and the lettuce looks a bit desiccated, so I don't want to harvest it until midday. With the warmth it will perk up as its leaves rehydrate. We replace the Agribon.

"Enrique, let's clean the snow off all the other hoop houses to see if we can get even bigger chunks of snow." Enrique loves that idea and we spend the rest of our time pulling snow off the hoops and comparing the size of snow chunks each of us cuts out.

After we get a hoop house cleared off, we look into each tunnel to see how our vegetables are doing. We are lucky, as the oakleaf lettuce, mizuna (*Brassica juncea* var. *japonica*), turnip greens (*Brassica rapa* subsp. *rapa*), spinach (*Spinacia oleracea*), Swiss chard (*Beta vulgaris* var. *vulgaris*), cauliflower (*Brassica oleracea* var. *botrytis*), and carrots (*Daucus carota* subsp. *sativus*) are thriving in their little hoop homes. While it is only thirty-five degrees, Enrique is now indifferent to the cold and we stay out working for nearly an hour.

By midday it is time to harvest with Ravi, as the plants have regained their moisture and are leafed out. The temperature is supposed to get as low as five degrees this night, and I believe that the lettuce and a few other crops may not be able to tolerate such a temperature change. Ravi is puzzled but pleased that we are going to be harvesting greens. He has good garden skills, so he will be very helpful in cutting the lettuce low, thus giving it a chance to grow back in early Spring. Ravi and I work side by side, chatting but focusing on harvesting the lettuce before it gets cold again.

Unexpectedly Ravi screams, "Look, I found a worm!" I don't believe him initially, but Ravi proves me wrong as he holds up a big fat earthworm. He soon finds two more. It is hard to believe that worms would be up and about at this time of year, but then it makes sense when I consider the micro-climate we have created and the fact that the soil is warm under my fingers. Within thirty minutes we harvest over three pounds of lettuce and leave the worms behind.

Since Ravi has done such a good job I tell him he can have a carrot as a snack. At first he doesn't believe that carrots are available, but thinking about it, he reconsiders his position and starts his search. He pokes his head under the Agribon shielding a row of vegetables and searches for his "perfect" carrot; he is successful as he pulls out a fairly large purple one. "You know, Ravi, if you leave the carrots in the ground over Winter, their starch turns to sugar and they get very sweet, just like a cookie." He is surprised and asks if we can leave a few carrots in the ground so he can try them throughout Winter and early Spring. I agree.

I had planned to finish harvesting the greens with my last student of the day, but he is unavailable. It becomes my job to get kale *(Brassica oleracea* var. *sabellica)* for Tracy, who wants to make kale chips for the students. If I have any time left, I can also harvest the mizuna.

Pulling the Agribon partially off the hoops around two o'clock, I feel a wave of heat emerge from the ground. I go down on all fours, stretching across the bed with the Agribon covering my head and torso. I don't want to expose more of the bed and greens to the elements than I must. I feel an interesting contrast between my warm head and hands within the Agribon cover and my cold backside and feet, still planted in the snow. As I cut the tender stems and the smell of cut kale and warm soil pours over me, I feel that I am not in the North in December.

My solace is fading quickly, however, as clouds separate the warming sun from me and a chill hits. The mizuna will soon start to desiccate from the cold, so I need to quicken my pace. Within an hour I harvest four pounds of kale and three pounds of mizuna.

School will be out next week and I won't come back to the Children's Garden until next year. Before I lock up, I inspect all the hoops. I notice some plastic clips, which hold the Agribon in place, are missing. I replace them with spares from the shed and use pieces of duct tape to repair a few holes that have emerged. I'm hoping there will be more to harvest in the New Year, but I am happy to spend one more day in the garden with my students before retreating into the greenhouse for much of the oncoming Winter.

INDEX OF PLANT NAMES

ABOUT THE AUTHOR

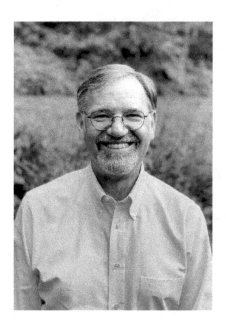

Erik Keller is a horticultural therapist and master gardener with 20-plus years of experience who has helped over 1,000 clients of all ages cope with physical, emotional, and mental challenges. He currently manages the gardens and horticultural therapy program at Ann's Place, Danbury, CT, an organization that assists cancer patients and their families. He is also a Conservation Commissioner in the town of Ridgefield, CT. He can be reached through Instagram @grohappy_ct or his website www.grohappy.com.

NOTE FROM THE AUTHOR

Word-of-mouth is crucial for any author to succeed. If you enjoyed *A Therapist's Garden*, please leave a review online—anywhere you are able. Even if it's just a sentence or two. It would make all the difference and would be very much appreciated.

Thanks!
Erik Keller

We hope you enjoyed reading this title from:

BLACK ROSE
writing™

www.blackrosewriting.com

Subscribe to our mailing list – *The Rosevine* – and receive
FREE books, daily deals, and stay current with news about
upcoming releases and our hottest authors.
Scan the QR code below to sign up.

Already a subscriber? Please accept a sincere thank you for
being a fan of Black Rose Writing authors.

View other Black Rose Writing titles at
www.blackrosewriting.com/books and use promo code
PRINT to receive a **20% discount** when purchasing.

CPSIA information can be obtained
at www.ICGtesting.com
Printed in the USA
BVHW051148020723
666681BV00006BA/368